Growing Older

Understanding quality of life in old age

Growing Older

Understanding quality of life in old age

edited by
Alan Walker

Open University Press

Open University Press
McGraw-Hill Education
McGraw-Hill House
Shoppenhangers Road
Maidenhead
Berkshire
England
SL6 2QL
email: enquiries@openup.co.uk
world wide web: www.openup.co.uk

and Two Penn Plaza, New York, NY 10121–2289, USA

First published 2005
Copyright © Alan Walker 2005

A catalogue record of this book is available from the British Library

ISBN 0335 21523 8 (pb) 0335 21524 6 (hb)

Library of Congress Cataloguing-in-Publication data
CIP data applied for

Typeset by RefineCatch Ltd, Bungay, Suffolk
Printed in Poland by OZGraf S.A. www.polskabook.pl

Contents

List of contributors

Sara Arber, Professor and Head of School of Human Sciences, Department of Sociology, University of Surrey
http://www.soc.surrey.ac.uk/sara_arber.htm

John Baldock, Professor of Social Policy and Dean of Social Sciences, University of Kent
http://www.kent.ac.uk/sspssr/staff/baldock.htm

Kate M. Bennett, Senior Lecturer, School of Psychology, University of Liverpool
http://www.liv.ac.uk/Psychology/Home.html

David Blane, Reader in Medical Sociology, Imperial College London
http://www.ic.ac.uk

Ann Bowling, Professor of Health Services Research, Department of Primary Care and Population Sciences, University College London
http://www.ucl.ac.uk/primcare-popsci/aps/

Elizabeth Breeze, Senior Lecturer, Department of Epidemiology and Public Health, University College, London
http://www.ucl.ac.uk/epidemiology

Jabeer Butt, Deputy Director, REU
http://www.reu.org.uk

Lynda Clarke, Course Director/Senior Lecturer, London School of Hygiene and Tropical Medicine
http://www.lshtm.ac.uk/cps/staff/lclarke.html

Peter G. Coleman, Professor of Psychogerontology, School of Psychology, University of Southampton
http://www.psychology.soton.ac.uk

Kate Davidson, Lecturer in Social Policy and Sociology, Department of Sociology and Co-Director of the Centre for Research on Ageing and Gender (CRAG), University of Surrey
http://www.soc.surrey.ac.uk/kate_davidson.htm

Murna Downs, Professor in Dementia Studies, Bradford Dementia Group, University of Bradford
http://www.brad.ac.uk/acad/health/bdg.htm

Maria Evandrou, Reader in Gerontology, Institute of Gerontology, King's College London
http://www.kcl.ac.uk/kis/schools/life_sciences/health/gerontology/index.php?pg=101

Ken Gilhooly, Professor of Psychology, School of Psychology, University of Hertfordshire
http://perseus.herts.ac.uk/uhinfo/schools/psy/research.cfm

Mary Gilhooly, Professor of Gerontology and Health Studies, Head of School of Social Work and Primary Care, University of Plymouth
http://www.plymouth.ac.uk/pages/dynamic.asp?page=staffdetails&id=mgilhooly

Jane Gow, Research Fellow, Institute for Applied Social and Health Research, School of Social Sciences, University of Paisley
http://www.paisley.ac.uk/socialscience/researchinstitute

Jan Hadlow, Senior Lecturer in Social Work, Canterbury Christ Church University College
http://health.cant.ac.uk/health-and-social/staff.htm

Catherine Hagan Hennessy, Professor of Public Health and Ageing, School of Social Work and Primary Care, University of Plymouth

Paul Higgs, Reader in Medical Sociology, Centre for Behavioural and Social Sciences in Medicine, University College London
http://www.ucl.ac.uk/medicine/behavioural-social/

Caroline Holland, Research Associate, Faculty of Health and Social Care, The Open University
http://www.open.ac.uk/shsw/

Georgina M. Hughes, Research Assistant, School of Psychology, University of Liverpool
http://www.liv.ac.uk/Psychology/Home.html

Martin Hyde, Research Fellow, Centre for Behavioural and Social Sciences in Medicine, University College London
http://www.ucl.ac.uk/medicine/behavioural-social/

Leonie Kellaher, Director of Centre for Environmental and Social Studies in Ageing (CESSA), London Metropolitan University
http://www.londonmet.ac.uk/pg-prospectus-2003/research/centres/cessa.cfm

Mary Maynard, Professor, Department of Social Policy and Social Work, University of York
http://www.york.ac.uk/depts/spsw/staff/maynard.html

Kevin McKee, Senior Lecturer, Sheffield Institute for Studies on Ageing, University of Sheffield
http://www.shef.ac.uk/sisa/Staff_McKee.shtml

Christopher McKevitt, Senior Research Fellow, Department of Public Health Sciences, King's College London
http://www.phs.kcl.ac.uk/stroke/

Fionnuala McKiernan, Programme Tutor, Doctoral Programme in Clinical Psychology, University of Southampton
http://psy.soton.ac.uk/

Marie Mills, Visiting Fellow, Centre for Research in Health Psychology, University of Southampton

Jo Moriarty, Research Fellow, Social Care Workforce Research Unit, King's College London
http://www.kcl.ac.uk

James Nazroo, Professor of Medical Sociology, University College London
http://www.ucl.ac.uk/medical-sociology

Sheila Peace, Associate Dean (Research) and Director of Research, Faculty of Health and Social Care, The Open University
http://www.open.ac.uk/shsw

Thomas Scharf, Reader in Social Gerontology and Director of the Centre for Social Gerontology, Keele University
http://www.keele.ac.uk/depts/so/csg/index.htm

Philip T. Smith, Professor, School of Psychology, University of Reading
http://www.personal.rdg.ac.uk/~sxsptsmi/home.html

Peter Speck, Visiting Fellow, Faculty of Medicine and Health Sciences, Southampton University
Pws7749@ntlworld.com

Susan Tester, Senior Lecturer in Social Policy, Department of Applied Social Science, University of Stirling
http://www.stir.ac.uk/Departments/HumanSciences/AppSocSci/SSP/staff/Stester.htm

Christina Victor, Professor of Social Gerontology and Health Services Research, School of Health and Social Care, University of Reading
http://www.rdg.ac.uk/health/staff/Victor.html

Alan Walker, Professor of Social Policy, Department of Sociological Studies, University of Sheffield, and Director of the ESRC Growing Older Programme
http://www.shef.ac.uk/socst/staff/a_walker.htm
http://www.shef.ac.uk/uni/projects/gop/

Peter Warr, Emeritus Professor, Institute of Work Psychology, University of Sheffield.
http://www.shef.ac.uk/~iwp

Lorna Warren, Lecturer, Department of Sociological Studies, University of Sheffield
http://www.shef.ac.uk/socst/staff/l_warren.htm

Dick Wiggins, Professor of Social Statistics and Director of the Sociology Research Methodology Centre, City University, London
http://www.staff.city.ac.uk/~sg399/

Fiona Wilson, Expert Patient Facilitator, Combined Universities of Sheffield Interprofessional Learning Unit, University of Sheffield and Hallam University
http://www.shef.ac.uk/cuilu/htm

Preface

This, the third introductory volume to the ESRC Growing Older (GO) Programme series, represents a unique undertaking whereby the researchers who carried out 22 of the 24 projects combined in thematic groups to synthesize their findings. The result is the most comprehensive account available in one place of the myriad findings from the GO Programme. The Programme context was the essential basis for this collective endeavour but so also was the goodwill of those involved. Coming at the end of the life of a Programme that had made many demands on them, it was remarkable that they responded so warmly to the proposal to put together this volume, indeed, their enthusiasm overcame my initial ambivalence in broaching the subject. First thanks therefore go to the collaborators in this book and, indeed, to all of the 96 researchers associated with the Programme. As well as a commemorative mug, they have my lasting thanks for being such a pleasure to work with.

Catherine Hagan Hennessy served for two years as Deputy Director on the Programme, though we worked as a team on all fronts. She was a truly excellent colleague and has my warmest personal thanks for all her help and support in the latter stages of the GO Programme, as well as in the detailed discussions involved in the planning of this volume.

The ESRC provided the funding for the GO Programme and, without that, there would be no research to report. But the ESRC's role extended far beyond funding. The Programme had excellent support from the ESRC, from within the Anthropology, Linguistics, Psychology, Health and Sociology Research Area led by Ros Rouse; from Kathy Ham and Iain Stewart of the External Relations Division; and from a series of ESRC programme officers, including Faye Auty and Naomi Beaumont, at the beginning, and Shabnam Khan, at the end.

It is essential to acknowledge on behalf of the 24 projects and the Programme as a whole, the thousands of older people who took part in the GO projects as respondents and sometimes researchers or who contributed to the Programme in other ways.

The Programme Advisory Committee, chaired by Anthea Tinker, was a constant source of support and my thanks go to its members: Allan Bowman, Gillian Crosby, Leela Damodaran, Arthur Fleiss, Tessa Harding, Tom Hoyes,

Paul Johnson, Carol Lupton, Robin Means, Terry Philpot, Martin Shreeve and Tony Warnes. Anthea Tinker could not have been a better chair in displaying a perfect balance of challenging questions and encouragement and in being a pleasure to work with. Arthur Fleiss was particularly helpful in creating links with policy-makers and Tessa Harding similarly with regard to NGOs working in the field of ageing. Shona Mullen and her colleagues at Open University Press have been extremely enthusiastic and supportive in the production of this and other volumes in the series.

Colleagues at the University of Sheffield have been very supportive towards the GO Programme, the Sheffield Institute for Studies on Ageing and the Department of Sociological Studies, especially Tim Booth, who helped to ensure that it was properly staffed and located. The amount of time and effort required to direct a research programme and to produce outputs such as this entails a heavy cost in terms of the time available for family life. Without the understanding and support of Carol Walker, it would have been impossible.

Last, but certainly not least, our sincere thanks go to the programme coordination team, including Alison Ball, Jo Levesley, Kristina Martimo and Roberta Nelson and, above all, to Marg Walker, for their major contributions to the whole GO Programme. Additional thanks and admiration go to Marg Walker for the efficiency she showed in the production of this volume.

Alan Walker
Department of Sociological Studies
University of Sheffield

1

Investigating quality of life in the growing older programme

Alan Walker and Catherine Hagan Hennessy

Introduction

The main purpose of this book is to synthesize the findings from the ESRC Growing Older (GO) Programme – the largest social science investigation of ageing and older people ever undertaken in the UK. Of course, it is impossible to include everything generated by 24 projects over a five-year period. Furthermore, to try to include a separate report on every project would mean simply duplicating the GO Findings series. Instead this book represents a unique undertaking whereby researchers from the different projects have come together and combined their findings under eight major themes. The outcome is a series of syntheses in which the GO researchers have successfully achieved the desired aims of informing readers about the specifics of their individual projects and drawing out the common threads in their results and policy/practice implications. This joint endeavour was planned at the final GO Programme meeting where opportunities were created for the proposed teams to prepare their initial outlines. Subsequently the teams worked together – a process that was facilitated greatly by their previous experience of being part of a unified research programme. Indeed, it is difficult to imagine this sort of combined effort being possible without an organized context such as this and, particularly, in the absence of funding for meetings. The fact that 22 out of 24 projects are represented here is remarkable and a real tribute to the commitment of the scientists involved.

This book is the third in the GO series and the last of the three edited volumes that provide an overview of the Programme (Walker and Hagan Hennessy 2004) and place it in a European context (Walker 2005a). As well as the GO Findings produced by every project and a summary booklet (Walker and Hennessy 2003), there is a CD-ROM containing all of the Programme's outputs (available from the Programme Office). Also the publications can be downloaded from the GO website (http://www.shef.ac.uk/uni/projects/gop/index.htm). However, this volume provides the most comprehensive report available on the key results of the GO Programme.

In the rest of this Introduction we provide an overview of the following chapters and the key themes of the Programme, summarize the different methodological approaches taken to the measurement of quality of life (QoL), and, first of all, outline the structure and operation of the GO Programme.

The GO Programme

The background and development of the Programme have been described in detail elsewhere (Walker 2004; Walker and Hagan Hennessy 2004). The first of the 24 separate projects comprising the Programme began in October 1999 and the last ended in April 2003. The Programme itself concluded at the end of July 2004. GO had two main objectives: (1) to create a multi-disciplinary and coordinated social science programme aimed at producing new knowledge on the factors that determine quality in later life; and (2) to try to contribute to the development of policies and practice so as to influence the extension of quality life.

While the extent to which the Programme achieved these objectives is a matter for independent assessment there is no doubt, first, that the Programme included a wide range of social science disciplines: anthropology, economics, education, psychology, social gerontology, social policy, social statistics and sociology. Second, it generated a vast body of new knowledge about QoL in old age, only a small fraction of which had been analysed and published at the time of writing. Avoiding a tedious list of the unique contributions of each project, for every one had something new to say about quality in later life, it includes the first representative study in the UK about what constitutes QoL for older people; the most comprehensive research so far on black and ethnic minority ageing; the first representative study on the impact of social exclusion on older people living in deprived areas; the first UK investigation of the pension implications of multiple role occupancy in mid-life; the first research on spiritual beliefs among bereaved spouses; a unique national survey of grandparenting and the first research on the successful ageing priorities of older women from different ethnic groups. In addition to producing a large amount of high quality new knowledge, the GO Programme made a substantial contribution to both quantitative and qualitative research methods, some important elements of which we return to below.

Third, there is no doubt that the Programme tried to transmit its findings to the worlds of policy and practice. A wide array of approaches was used to achieve this goal including the GO Findings series, linking projects to policy-makers, holding special seminars for policy-makers and practitioners and making presentations to policy/practice audiences. Whether or not the strategy adopted by the Programme has been successful in influencing policy and practice to the benefit of older people is a matter for retrospective evaluation but there are at least two grounds for optimism. On the one hand, it is clear that the findings from the projects have reached the hands of key policy-makers and some have been cited already and, on the other, media commentators have recognized the enormous potential of the Programme as an evidence base for policy and practice (Dean 2003) as have influential Quangos, including the Social Care Institute for Excellence. In addition, determined efforts were made by the GO Programme to involve older people in all aspects of its operation. This includes widespread dissemination of the findings, the centrepiece of which is a specially commissioned summary of the Programme by older people and for older people (Owen and Bell 2004). It is hoped that, armed with this information on what factors enhance or diminish the quality of later life, older people will be able to argue more effectively for changes in policy and practice.

A thematic approach to understanding quality of life

The GO Programme specification highlighted six broad topics:

+ Defining and measuring quality of life (5 projects)

+ Inequalities in quality of life (5 projects)

+ The role of technology and the built environment (2 projects)

+ Healthy and productive ageing (3 projects)

+ Family and support networks (6 projects)

+ Participation and activity in later life (3 projects).

These six topics effectively set the scientific agenda for the Programme and all of the original outline proposals fell within at least one of them. The spread of the 24 projects funded eventually can be seen above and their uneven distribution is explained by the bottom-up nature of the commissioning process. In drafting the specification, the main aim was to encourage research on those aspects of QoL in old age that had, thus far, received too little attention. The only topic that attracted insufficient outline proposals was technology and the built environment and neither of the two projects that were funded in this area concerned technology (their subjects were residential location and transport).

In practice, however, very few of the 24 projects could be confined easily to only one topic area, even the very broad ones above. Not surprisingly, as the projects developed and the Programme approach began to take effect, the overlaps and synergies between them became more and more apparent. This included instrument sharing, analytical cross-fertilization and common data collection. These overlaps were not a problem in any way because the original six topic areas were *a priori* construction designed to assist the commissioning process (including the primary aim of obtaining ESRC approval for the Programme itself). Thus, when it came to discussion of the themes for this volume, the original six topics were only one reference point. In this way, the danger of an artificial agenda being imposed upon the projects was avoided and what took place was an iterative process which was determined primarily by the scientific content of the projects and the common strands between them. In some cases joint working had already taken place, as a result of being part of the Programme, before the proposal was made for a thematic volume. The eight themes represented in Chapters 2–10 in fact are the ones we first proposed to the project teams but they were the results of successive rounds of discussion and, subsequently, there was significant traffic between themes. The eight themes are:

- Meaning and measurement of quality of life
- Inequalities in quality of life
- The environments of ageing
- Family and economic roles
- Social participation
- Social isolation and loneliness
- Frailty, identity and social support
- Bereavement.

It could be argued that social isolation and loneliness are part of the theme of social participation but combining them might downplay the significance both of the research findings reported here and the need for policies to combat these extreme forms of social exclusion. Alternatively, a more traditional approach to the topic of ageing might have chosen themes such as age, gender and ethnicity but, in the GO Programme, these were horizontal themes running through many projects to a greater or lesser extent.

Of course, there is a risk that our collective approach to the quality of later life is determined by the GO Programme's agenda. This must be true in the broad sense that we have considered only the social science aspects of this issue. Within that boundary, however, the authors of this volume have emphasized other topics not covered by the Programme where they consider this to be necessary. As a result, what is presented in the subsequent chapters is the most comprehensive assessment available of QoL in old age. We are not claiming that every single aspect of quality in later life is covered, indeed, there are obvious gaps such as the role of technology, pensions policy, the global political economy of ageing, comparative analyses (but see Walker 2005a), and the ageing of people with learning difficulties. Nonetheless, the eight themes that are represented in this volume cover the great majority of issues concerning quality in later life.

The first theme is the meaning and measurement of QoL. As mentioned already, the GO Programme can claim to have progressed substantially the conceptualization and measurement of QoL in old age, especially with regard to approaches which articulate older people's own perspectives on its nature and constituent elements. In the next section we review the various methods employed by GO researchers to measure QoL. In Chapter 2, covering this topic, Ken Gilhooly, Mary Gilhooly and Ann Bowling begin with an outline of the long history of interest in happiness and well-being stretching back to the fourth century BC. They show how, more recently, the concept of QoL has emerged with a public policy engine behind it. Drawing on the experiences of various GO projects, this chapter examines the complex issues associated with measuring QoL. Its main focus is psychometric issues such as the processes involved in answering the most common QoL questions asked by researchers.

The second theme also represents one of the major contributions to the literature by the GO Programme: inequalities in QoL. This theme formed part of the original specification for the Programme because of the enduring salience of one of the key messages from the original formulations of the political economy of ageing perspective that the material circumstances experienced by different groups of older people are largely the result of the roles and statuses they occupied at previous stages of the lifecourse; with employment status and socio-economic class being particularly influential (Dowd 1980; Walker, 1980, 1981; Minkler and Estes 1984; Guillemard 1984). The emphasis on the life-course in this perspective has proved to be particularly influential. More recently social gerontologists have highlighted the significance of gender, which was part of the original conception, and ethnicity which was not (Arber and Ginn 1991, 1995; Blakemore and Boneham 1994; Modood et al. 1997).

Chapter 3 concerns the inequalities theme and draws on the results of four GO projects. Paul Higgs and his six-co-authors stress the need to understand inequalities as more than a simple absence of something. They first consider socio-economic disadvantage among older people and report its strong corre-lations with poor health, functioning and morale in old age. For example, those in social classes IV and V living in council or housing association rented accommodation are more than twice as likely to report a mobility problem than those from social classes I and II who own their property. This analysis confirms the political economy of ageing thesis that older people do not escape the legacy of their earlier socio-economic history and, at the same time, it reinforces a second key message from this perspective that policy action may exacerbate or ameliorate disadvantage. The need for action to reduce health inequalities is stressed in this chapter. The analysis of the interaction of gender and marital status shows the continuation of strikingly wide inequalities in old age. For example, the risk of having a low household income in later life is nearly five times as great for divorced women than for married men. While divorced men may be more disadvantaged financially than other men, their income is much higher than that of divorced women. Again this research points to the influence of both individual lifecourses and the impact of social processes which create the contexts for QoL.

The consideration of ethnic inequalities in the quality of later life reveals the major gap between those in ethnic minority groups and their white contempo-raries. These differences are particularly marked in the areas of income and wealth, housing conditions and health. Importantly too, this analysis demon-strates divergencies *among* ethnic minority groups as well as between them and the white majority. The fourth component of this chapter is inequalities in early old age. In common with the other studies, this one shows the importance of a lifecourse perspective. In particular it emphasizes the accumulation of dis-advantages over the lifecourse at home and at work and their negative impact on the quality of later life. However, when these accumulated disadvantages are analysed alongside present-day factors, the latter were shown to exert the most powerful effects on QoL. But, as the authors acknowledge, the distinction between current and lifecourse factors is artificial to some extent because the latter are implicit in many of the former.

The fundamental role of the environment – social, cultural, economic and physical – in creating opportunities for or barriers to QoL was emphasized by a variety of GO projects and not only the two originally classified under this theme. It was the priority given to contextualizing QoL by the Programme which resulted in the environment emerging as such a significant factor to the quality of later life. Chapter 4 covers this theme using the results of four projects. The seven authors argue that 'environment' is not a unitary experience but a series of settings in which daily life takes place. The chapter argues that getting out and about is a fundamental QoL issue. For example, in both rural and urban areas, having to stay at home for health reasons increases by nearly three times the chances of having poor morale. The chapter also considers the importance of neighbourhood, social contact, transport and security and, by combining the results of the four studies, is able to provide a rich picture of the importance of a range of material, social and psychological aspects of the environments of old age. The chapter ends with a plea to policy-makers to recognize the importance of opportunities to get out and about.

The fourth theme, like the second, reflects the political economy theoretical paradigm in highlighting the critical importance of family and work roles in determining the material circumstances of old age. But the discussion of family and economic roles in Chapter 5 extends that approach in two respects: on the one hand, it stresses the importance of family roles for well-being in later life and, on the other, it broadens the analysis of economic roles to include a consideration of their desirability to the incumbent. The three authors succinctly describe the theoretical background to their research covering multiple roles, commitments, the significance of family roles and intergenerational exchanges. The starting point for their analysis is the centrality of family relations to well-being and it uses the results of the GO study of grandparenthood to emphasize this point. The overwhelming significance of relations with grandchildren is clear from the GO research: over 80 per cent of grandparents say it contributes a lot (31 per cent) or enormously (55 per cent) to their QoL. Then they discuss the key role of paid employment and, specifically, the impact on well-being of different employment statuses. The older unemployed are the most deprived but there are no overall differences in well-being or life satisfaction between older people who have a job and the retired. The authors stress that QoL is influenced not by the role incumbency itself but by two other sets of factors: the nature of the environment that is experienced and a

7

person's wish to be in that environment. Finally, the combination of family and economic roles is analysed. Here the focus is on 'parent', 'carer' and 'paid worker' roles. The combination of family and economic roles over the life-course is a much more common occurrence than at any one point in time. The penalty that many women carry for fulfilling the important roles of carers and parents is reliance on low means-tested incomes in old age.

The fifth theme, participation, formed part of the original GO specification because of the relative absence of research on this topic in the UK, particularly with regard to variations based on gender and ethnicity. The discussion of social involvement in Chapter 6 is based on the results of three projects. While welcoming the recent expansion of information on the social contacts of older people, from national surveys such as the General Household Survey (GHS) and the English Longitudinal Survey of Ageing (ELSA), the three authors question the methodological capacity of such surveys to understand the nature of social participation. On the basis of their qualitative investigations the authors illustrate the factors that enhance and limit the extent and quality of social involvement with a specific focus on age, gender and ethnicity. The chapter reports significant differences in social involvement by older men depending on their partnership status, with older divorced and never married men having the most restricted networks of kin, friends and neighbours. Then it highlights the importance of family and extended networks in the lives of women from minority ethnic groups and the centrality of community and belonging. Finally, the chapter reports that individual spiritual resources play an important part in older women's lives.

In Chapter 7 Christina Victor and Thomas Scharf consider the converse of social participation, social isolation and loneliness. First of all, they outline the general patterns of social and civic engagement among older people as a back-ground to their discussion of isolation and loneliness. Both projects represented in this chapter show that older people maintain high levels of contact with a range of people including neighbours, friends and family, although the level of contact with neighbours is slightly lower in the deprived areas studied by Scharf and his colleagues. The two research studies also demonstrate high levels of involvement of older people in community life. For example, three-quarters of respondents in England's most deprived areas had undertaken at least one type of civic activity in the past three years. Using a specially constructed relative social isolation index, the data are compared and this reveals greater levels of medium to high isolation among older people in the national survey (36 per cent) compared with those living in deprived areas

(20 per cent). In both studies, although different approaches to assessing it were taken, severe loneliness was experienced by only a minority of respondents. Although differences were found in overall levels of loneliness between the two studies, the reasons for which are discussed, both studies link loneliness with marital status and, specifically, they highlight the vulnerability of widowed older people. This echoes the findings reported in Chapter 3 on inequalities in QoL and pre-empts the analysis in Chapter 9.

The seventh theme is the impact of frailty on the quality of later life and the strategies older people employ to maintain their identity when faced with physical and cognitive decline. The findings of three GO projects form the empirical basis of Chapter 8: McKee et al.'s (2002) study of reminiscence among frail older people; Tester et al.'s (2003) research on perceptions of QoL of frail older people; and Gilhooly et al.'s (2003) project on cognitive functioning. Although the three projects took different approaches to frailty and its impact, there are common themes in their findings. For example, discontinuity and loss were experienced by frail older people in the loss of their home, friends and familiar company, their decline in physical health or cognitive functioning, in feeling cut off in the present world or indifferent to fellow residents in a care or nursing home. More positively, various strategies were used to counteract such discontinuities, including having a significant role in the family, keeping active and sustaining cognitive functioning, all of which are aimed at maintaining continuity of identity. A key role is played by communication, for example, in building and sustaining relationships through reminiscence and through participation in meaningful activities.

Chapter 9 continues the theme of frailty and identity combining the results of three projects on the role of social support services. All three studies found that the use of care services was mediated through the key activities of maintaining and reconstructing identities and social relationships following increasing dependence and reliance on help from other people. The projects concerned stroke patients, frail housebound older people and older people from different ethnic groups. All of them illustrate that loss of independence necessitates identity work in order to sustain conceptions of self, and that adjustments are made often with major improvements. However, the older people in these studies did not usually see professional service providers as a potential source of improvement. It was increased contact with others that was most likely to raise self-esteem. The studies also reveal considerable divergence between older people's conceptions of their circumstances and needs and those of service providers. It is not that either side is mistaken but their perspectives are necessarily different.

Bereavement, the eighth theme, was mentioned in the original GO specification but it was not one of the six main themes. It emerged within the Programme because it was the focus of two projects which researched the experiences of older bereaved spouses. In Chapter 10 Peter Speck and his six co-authors begin by outlining the various models of bereavement. Then they focus on the results of the two projects, one an exploratory study based on a series of individual case studies into the role of spiritual beliefs following bereavement and the other an investigation of the influence of gender and widowhood on well-being in later life. The former found clear associations between spiritual beliefs and well-being following bereavement and, while the latter was not specifically concerned with religious belief, the findings revealed that it did play a significant role for some respondents by providing meaning to their lives following the death of their spouse. The chapter also looks at some of the methodological issues encountered by the two teams in researching this sensitive topic.

We have already noted the impossibility of including references to every contributory factor to QoL in old age and every finding from the GO projects. Nonetheless the authors of the thematic chapters have succeeded in both making their project findings accessible and in synthesizing the common elements between projects in order to further our understanding of what constitutes quality in later life.

Methodological approaches in measuring quality of life

In commissioning projects on a broad range of aspects of QoL in old age, the Programme explicitly set out to chart the territory of QoL beyond the traditional borders of its health-related dimensions. As described above, a hallmark of the Programme was an expanded conceptualization of QoL that drew directly on older people's perspectives regarding its nature and constituent factors, encompassing less recognized dimensions and reflecting a rejection of the social construction of later life as being essentially problematic. Accordingly, the programme projects were characterized by a high degree of methodological diversity, and mixed quantitative and qualitative methods were frequently used to provide objective indicators of QoL as well as to capture the subjective or 'insider's' viewpoint of the older person concerning what gave value and meaning to their lives.

The majority (18 out of 24) of the GO projects used some form of mixed methods design with the remainder employing either quantitative (3) or qualitative (3) methods only. Consistent with the mainstreaming of qualitative approaches in gerontological research to understand and explain complex issues (Cobb and Forbes 2002), among the projects making use of qualitative methods, a wide range of techniques was employed: observation, in-depth interviewing, focus groups, free-listing, personal diaries, and innovative projective instruments. Tester and her colleagues (2003), for example, utilized multiple ethnographic methods to investigate how frail older residents – many with communication difficulties due to speech, hearing and cognitive impairments – define and realize QoL within the confines of a care home setting. These included observation, structured group discussions, in-depth interviews, and in the case of residents with impaired communication, the use of a novel tool ('Talking Mats') which is based on the non-verbal elicitation of preferences. This particular project represents a watershed in research on the QoL of older people in that it overcame a host of assumptions and challenges about the possibility of empirically investigating QoL among those who are unable to verbally express their views. Indeed, this and many of the other GO projects transcended previous conventional approaches used to assess QoL in gerontological research based on what has been referred to as 'the law of the easily measurable' (Hennessy and Hennessy 1990). Yet another example of an inclusive research approach used in the GO Programme that was aimed at directly tapping older women's QoL experiences was the participatory action research conducted by Cook et al. (2003) which closely involved research participants throughout the project in designing and carrying out the research and helping to interpret the study findings.

Researchers also used a variety of analytic strategies to make sense of the massive volume of qualitative data collected in the GO projects. While some of these strategies were more inductively orientated and aimed at building theory grounded in the data (for example, life history approach, narrative analysis, content analysis), others such as the framework analysis (Ritchie and Spencer 1993) used by Nazroo and his colleagues (2003) were more deductively orientated and intended to answer comparatively focused questions regarding QoL. Collectively, this rich toolkit of qualitative methods and approaches was employed to capture dynamic, experiential aspects of older people's QoL and to better characterize its content and context.

Among the projects employing quantitative data on QoL, several conducted secondary analysis of existing national survey data-sets. These data sources included, for example, the Health Survey for England, the General Household Survey, the British Household Panel Study, the Family and Working Lives

Study, the Retirement Survey and the Fourth National Survey of Ethnic Minorities. Two unique studies employed archival survey data to follow up historical cohorts (the 1937/39 Boyd-Orr Study and the 1972 Paisley-Renfrew 'MIDSPAN' Epidemiological Study), and a third drew data from an ongoing (unrelated) large-scale clinical trial. Still other projects conducted primary research on large nationally representative survey samples, for example, through the National Omnibus Survey. A number of the studies using data from national samples subsequently used them to draw theoretically-based purposive samples for qualitative interviewing.

The scope of the survey instruments used to measure QoL in the GO Programme was wide and reflected the breadth of the dimensions being researched. Many of the projects made use of standard QoL instruments (for example, the Sickness Impact Profile, Philadelphia Geriatric Morale Scale, SF-36, SEIQOL, WHO-QOL, LEIPAD, and Delighted–Terrible Faces Scale), while one (Blane et al. 2002) developed a new 19-item measure (CASP-19) emphasizing the ability to satisfy personal needs for control, autonomy, self-realization and pleasure (see Chapters 2 and 3). A number of the GO projects also tested measures of QoL with groups such as ethnic minority older people for whom the content validity of many existing QoL scales had not previously been established. Examples of the psychometric issues involved in the quantitative measurement of QoL that were encountered by GO researchers are discussed in Chapter 2 by Ken Gilhooly, Mary Gilhooly and Ann Bowling.

The methods and measures brought to bear on investigations of QoL in the GO projects were extremely diverse and typically involved hybrid approaches to mapping the expanded conception of QoL – both objective and subjective – underlying the GO Programme. Many of the projects that collected qualitative and quantitative data employed analytic strategies that involved using one type of data to reciprocally generate and explore hypotheses with the other type, thus enriching and cross-validating the findings. Most of the studies were based on cross-sectional designs, and therefore limited in their ability to capture the dynamic nature of QoL over time. However, these findings have produced baseline data for a multitude of research questions to be explored further in longitudinal studies.

Conclusion

Finally, the factors and processes relevant to QoL identified across the GO studies can be usefully summarized within Renwick and Brown's (1996) framework which consists of three primary dimensions of QoL termed 'being', 'belonging' and 'becoming'. 'Being' refers to the physical, psychological and spiritual aspects of QoL; 'belonging' is concerned with the adequacy of an individual's interpersonal relationships and their physical, social and community environments; while 'becoming' encompasses personal aspirations regarding purposeful activity, instrumental activity, leisure pursuits and personal growth (Nolan et al. 2001).

Taken as a whole, the findings from the GO Programme underscore the nature of QoL in older age as inherently multidimensional, dynamic, actively constructed with reference to past and present selves, and context-dependent. In other words, they tend to support those theoretical constructions of ageing which emphasize the reflexive interaction between individual and social structure over the lifecourse: the variable exercise of agency within social inclusion. The GO Programme provides a rich test bed for different theoretical approaches to ageing and older people as well as providing a launch pad for further empirical research on the quality of later life. The Programme's findings also provide substantial guidance for policy-makers and practitioners on a wide range of big (expensive) and small (inexpensive) interventions that could help to transform older people's lives. (The question as to whether or not policy and other action will follow from the findings of the GO projects is discussed in the final chapter.) It is the sincere hope of everyone involved in the GO Programme that those with the power to take such actions will respond to this challenge.

2

Quality of life
Meaning and measurement

Mary Gilhooly, Ken Gilhooly and Ann Bowling

Introduction

The dictionary definition of 'quality' is 'grade of goodness' (*Chambers Twentieth Century Dictionary* 1961). Mendola and Pelligrini (1979) defined quality of life (QoL) as 'the individual's achievement of a satisfactory social situation within the limits of perceived physical capacity'. Shin and Johnson (1978) defined QoL as 'the possession of resources necessary to the satisfaction of individual needs, wants and desires, participation in activities enabling personal development and self actualisation and satisfactory comparison between oneself and others'. More recently, the World Health Organization Quality of Life Group (1993) defined QoL as including the individual's perception of his or her position in life in the context of the culture and value systems in which they live and in relation to goals.

These various definitions reveal not only the complexity of the concept, but very real differences in opinion as to the nature of QoL. Like those before us, the researchers in the Growing Older (GO) Programme have struggled with both the conceptualization and measurement of QoL. The GO Programme did not impose any particular perspective (Walker 2001) and, as a consequence, a variety of different approaches were taken, reflecting possibly the personal orientations of the GO programme researchers (Tester et al. 2001). For example, Hyde et al. (2001), in describing their approach to the theory and properties of QoL, note that many writers on the topic have conflated influences on QoL with QoL. In their study of inequalities in QoL in early old age, an attempt was made to ensure that their measure of QoL was different from the things that might influence QoL (Blane et al. 2002). The perspective of

QoL developed for the Blane et al. study was derived from an explicit theory of human need which recognizes the social and biological as equal components with its 'needs satisfaction' approach. On the other hand, in both her study on transport and ageing (M. Gilhooly et al. 2002) and her study on cognitive functioning (M. Gilhooly et al. 2002), Gilhooly and her colleagues took an entirely pragmatic view and defined QoL as 'what our chosen measures measure' (Gilhooly 2001).

In this chapter we shall first examine QoL in relation to other related concepts, namely, happiness and well-being. Having considered the meaning of QoL, we then go on to examine issues associated with measuring QoL, wherever possible comparing and contrasting findings from studies in the GO Programme with other published literature.

Our examination of the measurement of QoL will focus largely on psychometric issues. There is, however, considerable debate about whether QoL can be measured at all, and whether it can be measured objectively, rather than merely tapping into subjective views. We do not intend to consider the objective/subjective debate in detail. This issue was considered in Gabriel and Bowling's chapter in the first book in the Growing Older Series, *Growing Older: Quality of Life in Old Age* (Walker and Hennessy 2004) and many of the GO programme researchers have written about the issue either in their reports or in subsequent journal articles (for example, McKee et al. 2002; Higgs et al. 2003; Hyde et al. 2003). Instead, our aim is to extend the expanding literature from the GO Programme by considering measurement issues which have yet to be explored in publications from the GO Programme.

Quality of life

Meanings

Interest in QoL is not a recent phenomenon (Chung et al. 1997). The Greek philosophers were much taxed by notions of happiness and the good life. Aristippus, a philosopher of the fourth century BC, taught that the goal of life is to experience the maximum amount of pleasure and that happiness is the sum total of hedonic episodes. Others in the hedonic tradition include Hobbes, who argued that happiness lies in the pursuit and fulfilment of human appetites and DeSade who argued that the pursuit of pleasure and sensation is the ultimate goal in life (Ryan and Deci 2001). More recently, psychologists such as Kubovy (1999) have argued that hedonism includes the pleasures and preferences of the mind as well as the body.

Aristotle believed that hedonic happiness was a vulgar ideal and argued that true happiness is found in doing what is worth doing (Ryan and Deci 2001). The term *eudaimonia* (*daimon* = true self) refers to this type of well-being. *Eudaimonia*, according to Waterman (1993), occurs when activities are congruent with deeply held values and are holistically engaged. Self-determination theory (Ryan and Deci 2000) has embraced the concept of *eudaimonia* as central to well-being. Ryff and Singer (1998, 2000), in their lifespan theory of human flourishing, argue that psychological well-being is distinct from subjective well-being, with psychological well-being tapping aspects of human actualization.

The ancient debate between hedonic and eudaimonic theorists continues to exert an influence on conceptions of well-being. However, what appears to have happened over the past 20 years is a move away from measures of, as well as interest in, the construct of well-being to discourse about 'quality of life'. There are a number of factors that have contributed to this change in discourse, as well as research interest. First, in medicine there was a need to recognize that many treatments and interventions could not cure disease, but could at best control unpleasant symptoms. For example, coronary artery bypass surgery could not cure heart disease, nor could it necessarily prevent a heart attack, but it could reduce the pain associated with angina. With reductions in angina pain, patients would be able to live a more normal and independent life, and would be less miserable. In other words, patients would be happier, not only because of a reduction in unpleasant events, but because they could engage in activities leading to self-actualization. However, an increase in 'happiness' (or reduction in unhappiness) probably did not sound like a very scientific health-related outcome, while improved 'quality of life' sounded far more objective as an outcome measure when assessing the impact of treatment and intervention. Not only did QoL appear to be an outcome with more scientific nuances, but it was, and perhaps still widely is, believed to be something that can be assessed by others, rather than relying on the subjective views of the patient.

A second factor contributing to the shift from a research interest in well-being to QoL over the past 20 years is a growing interest in inequalities in health, social exclusion and government policies that might disadvantage large sections of the population. Governments do not, on the whole, view themselves as responsible for individual happiness, but have come to acknowledge that there are things that governments can do to affect the quality of housing, the work and neighbourhood environments, and other things outside family and private life. It is convenient for governments to pool all of these into a general construct called 'quality of life', something which governments aim to improve, while at the same time arguing that not only is there little that they can do to ensure that such improvements ensure that individuals are happier or experience higher psychological well-being, but that it would be inappropriate for governments to intervene directly in family and personal life. Thus, QoL came to prominence as a concept as government departments set out programme evaluation. As in medicine, QoL proved to be a useful concept in that governments were unlikely to 'cure' many of the problems besetting society, but might be able to make improvements to the life quality of their population.

Although it is widely acknowledged that there is no one definition of QoL (Smith 2001), what seems to be clear is that there is a general reluctance to suggest that QoL is identical to hedonic happiness or *eudaimonia*. This may be because there is a growing body of literature suggesting that happiness and psychological well-being are related to personality characteristics which are not only stable across the life span, but which are biologically determined (Diener 2000). The personality characteristics most consistently and strongly related to subjective well-being are extraversion and neuroticism. Optimism and self-esteem are correlated with subjective well-being, though the direction of causality has not been determined. Temperament models of the relationship between personality and well-being posit that there are biological 'set points' of emotional experiences, that there are biological determinants for emotional reactions to stimuli, and/or that those with certain personalities are able to wrest more rewards from the environment (Diener and Lucas 1999).

If personality traits influence levels of subjective well-being, then there is little, or certainly less, that governments (or at least those in affluent liberal democracies) can do to increase well-being, hence the interest in the construct of QoL, rather than happiness or psychological well-being. What can, however, be hoped for by policy-makers is that policy can alter the environment, service provision, distribution of wealth, and so on, and that such factors will influence perceptions of QoL. The level of happiness or subjective well-being that results will, however, be determined, it could be argued, by individual personality traits.

Physical health will, of course, have a major impact on perceptions of QoL. However, in recent years it has been argued that government policies have a major impact on the likelihood of poor health. It is through their influence on levels of poverty and the distribution of wealth and status that government policies, it is argued, can influence health. Apart from influences on physical health, money itself may impact on perceptions of QoL, though the research evidence, especially in wealthy nations, is complex. While many would deny that money could buy them happiness, if asked, 'Would a little more money make you a little happier?' many will say yes (Myers 2000). A University of Michigan survey asking, 'What would improve your QoL?' revealed that 'more money' was the most frequent response (Campbell 1981). Studies comparing nations fairly consistently reveal that where low income threatens basic human needs, being relatively well off predicts greater well-being. However, where gross national product is more than $8,000 per person, the correlation between national wealth and well-being evaporates (Myers 2000). The picture is also complicated by the fact that wealth, civil rights, literacy and years of democracy are confounded. Studies of individuals have also revealed that very rich Americans are only slightly happier than the average American. The overall conclusion drawn by Myers (2000), when reviewing the relationship between money and happiness, is that happiness depends less on exterior things than might be expected. Indeed, as noted by Ryan and Deci (2001), several studies have indicated that the more people focus on financial and materialistic goals, the lower their well-being.

If happiness is completely subjective, little influenced by exterior factors such as money, and might even be biologically determined via personality traits, in what ways is QoL similar or different? As noted above, the growing interest in altering or influencing QoL, suggests a wide-spread belief that QoL is less subjective than happiness. However, in recent years there has been an increasing recognition that the evaluation of QoL is dependent on the person who experiences it (Benner 1985; Bowling 1997). In addition, QoL has increasingly been defined in specific domains, for example, health-related QoL, as well as in relation to specific illnesses, for example, Asthma Quality of Life Measure, Diabetes Quality of Life Questionnaire (McKee et al. 2002). Whether this is due to developments in measurement driving the conceptual work or vice versa is unclear. And because a high proportion of the QoL measures consider a range of domains of life – health, employment, relationships, and environment – it appears that the core notion of QoL is one of degree of satisfaction over all areas of life important for the individual concerned. Interestingly, this sounds rather more like *eudaimonia* than hedonic happiness.

It may, of course, be that QoL consists of both *eudaimonia* and hedonic happiness. Blane et al. (2002) conceptualized QoL as consisting of the satisfaction of needs in four areas: (1) control – the need to be able to act freely in one's environment; (2) autonomy – the need to be free from the undue interference of others; (3) self-realization – the need for self-realization; and (4) pleasure – the need to enjoy oneself. Thus, these GO programme researchers propose that QoL consists of both hedonic happiness (pleasure) and what could be taken as important elements of *eudaimonia*, namely control, autonomy and, central to *eudaimonia*, self-realization.

Measurement

Far more has been written about the measurement than about the concept of QoL. This may be because, even if it is difficult to define, most people feel that they know what is meant when the term 'quality of life' is used. However, what will be obvious from the following brief review of measurement is that there is a vast range of methods and that some serious and difficult issues arise when setting about measuring QoL.

Answering Quality of Life questions: possible processes

Quality of life research depends totally on individuals being able to respond to often rather complex and/or vague questions such as 'How satisfied are you with your life as a whole these days? Very satisfied, satisfied, not satisfied, not at all satisfied'. How do people tackle such questions? Does one maintain an internal 'mental meter' of subjective well-being from which a value can be read and mapped onto the satisfaction scale given in the questionnaire item? As we will see, this view cannot be sustained since responses are susceptible to a wide range of contextual factors. Rather, it appears that responses are constructed 'on-line' or 'on the fly' by using information that comes to mind at the time the question is encountered. The fact that test–retest reliability for subjective well-being is often low (0.4 to 0.6), even within a one-hour gap, is indicative of the importance of context effects. In their transport study, M. Gilhooly and her colleagues reported a test–retest retest reliability of 0.74, a figure that might be acceptable for some purposes, but which indicates that context effects might have been impacting on QoL judgements. Another example is that minor events, such as finding a small value coin or variations in order of questions can markedly affect responses (Schwartz 1987; Schwartz and Strack 1991). In addition, as reported by Beaumont and Kenealy (2003: 1), their GO project revealed that 'Reports of perceptions of QoL are heavily influenced by the nature of the question being asked.'

Accessibility

A typical QoL item might be 'Taking all things together, how would you say things are these days?' In the qualitative component of their GO study on QoL measurement, Bowling and Gabriel (2004) asked, 'First of all, thinking about your life as a whole, what is it that makes your life good – that is, the things that give your life quality?' In answering such a question people cannot systematically and exhaustively review all aspects of their lives to form an integrated representation and derive an overall judgement. Rather, people will tend to retrieve what they judge to be sufficient information on which to base an answer. In doing so they are relying on the information that is readily accessible to them in the time available to answer the question. *Accessibility* of information depends on the *recency* with which the information has been previously accessed and the *frequency* with which it has been accessed. For example, if one has been very recently reminded of a pleasant childhood experience that information will be readily accessible and thus may enter a judgement about satisfaction with one's life as a whole. Or, one may be dwelling frequently on a particular problem at work that would be highly accessible and, hence, likely to enter into a process of judging current life satisfaction.

A number of experimental studies have demonstrated effects of accessibility on life satisfaction and well-being judgements. For example, Strack et al. (1988) asked undergraduate students questions about dating frequency and about general life satisfaction. They found that if the dating question came second then the correlation between dating frequency and life satisfaction was a non-significant –0.12. However, if the dating question was placed before the life satisfaction question, then the correlation between dating and life satisfaction became a substantial 0.66. Similar results have been found for other groups when the questions concerned marital satisfaction and life satisfaction. If the marital satisfaction question came first the two items correlated highly; if it came second, the items were much less correlated (Schwartz et al. 1991). The interpretation of these results is that a preceding question (e.g., dating frequency) brings information to mind that would not otherwise be used in making the overall life satisfaction judgement. Thus, conclusions about the role of dating in undergraduate life satisfaction could vary dramatically depending on the order of questions being asked (because order affects accessibility through a recency effect).

Lest readers think that these studies are irrelevant to assessing QoL in old age, it is worth noting that in their GO transport and ageing study, M. Gilhooly and her colleagues (2002) found that overall QoL ratings were much higher, indeed, markedly skewed to the positive end of the scale, when QoL was rated before ratings of the quality of public transport. Asking study participants to first rate the quality of bus, train and underground travel brought about a more 'normal' distribution of responses on the Delighted–Terrible Faces rating scale of overall QoL. Although it was thought that this reduction in skew was due to getting study participants to think about their QoL as something more 'external' to themselves, it could be that prior negative thoughts about difficulties of using public transport influenced thoughts about overall QoL.

Using accessible information: assimilation, contrast and duration effects

Retrieved information about the same event may have contrary effects depending on how the information is used. For example, a negative event, if recent, will likely be *assimilated* into a judgement of 'my life now' and so reduce reported satisfaction; but, if the negative event was not recent, it may form a *contrast* with the current state of affairs and so lead to a boosting of currently reported satisfaction. Thus, Elder (1974) found that older people in the USA who had been young in the Great Depression generally reported higher subjective well-being the more they had suffered poor economic conditions as teenagers. Another contrast effect was observed by Runyan (1980) who found that upwardly mobile people remembered childhood as less satisfactory than downwardly mobile individuals, presumably by contrast with their current circumstances.

In assessing extended episodes it appears that people tend to make particular use of affective peaks and the affective value of the end stage of the event. Kahneman et al. (1993) reported intuitively surprising results that people who underwent an unpleasant medical procedure preferred longer periods of discomfort to shorter periods if the end stage was a gradual drop in discomfort as against an abrupt change. So, in some circumstances, more pain is preferred to less! Information about duration of the painful episodes seems to be neglected. Peak levels of pain were also influential in judging preferences for such episodes. Overall, judgements of pain seem to follow a 'peak and end' heuristic which only takes these two aspects into account. Similar patterns have also been found in judgements of pleasant episodes using films as stimuli (Kahneman et al. 1993). Thus, the effects of a three-year negative period (for example, being unemployed) on overall life satisfaction may not be much more than that of a shorter period in the long run, given use of the 'peak and end' heuristic which ignores duration. Also, a prolonged positive period may be reduced in subjective value by a brief downturn at the end.

Mood states

Affective feelings at the time that QoL judgements are made can affect responses. For example, being tested in a pleasant room or when the sun is

21

shining have been shown to affect subjective well-being judgements (Schwartz and Clore 1983; Schwartz 1987). Why might these results occur? One possibility is that current and very recent events strongly influence moods which in turn increase accessibility of mood congruent information. People in a happy mood more readily retrieve happy memories and those in a sad mood more readily retrieve sad memories. Hence the accessible information that goes into the judgement process is congruent with prevailing mood and will affect judgements accordingly. A second route is that the mood itself may be used as a quick basis for responding. That is, one can apply a 'mood heuristic', that is, 'If I feel good at this moment, it is likely that my life is generally good.' Thus, an answer can very quickly be given to a general QoL question without extensive cognitive processing of relevant information. Indeed, when Ross et al. (1986) asked participants to explain their life satisfaction judgements, a majority referred to their current affective state saying, for example, 'Well, I feel good.'

It seems likely that use of the 'mood heuristic' would tend to occur with the more cognitively demanding questions regarding an overall assessment since the heuristic offers a low effort short-cut. It would be less likely when the questions are more domain-specific. Schwartz (1987) found that the results of a football game important to the participants affected their overall life satisfaction responses but not their satisfaction judgements regarding the more specific domains of work and income.

Reporting and editing

In reporting levels of general life satisfaction, happiness, well-being, and QoL, there is scope for the operation of social desirability effects. Self-reported QoL levels are typically quite high. In a survey and recalibration of a large number of studies from across the world involving some 1.1 million participants, Myers and Diener (1996) found that the average rated happiness was nearly 7 on a 0–10-point scale where 0 was very unhappy, 5 was neutral and 10 was the high extreme. A large study using the Faces scale in Detroit (Andrews and Withey 1976) found that 90 per cent picked one of the happy faces as representing how they felt about their lives as a whole. Similarly, Gilhooly et al. (2002, 2003) in a study on mid-life risk factors for declines in cognitive functioning in old age carried out under the GO Programme found that 89 per cent of their sample of 145 older people chose one of the happy faces to represent their current QoL. Likewise, in their GO study on transport and QoL, Gilhooly and her colleagues (2002) found that ratings on the faces scales of QoL were skewed toward the 'delighted' end of the scale. In another GO project, Bowling and Gabriel (2004) reported that almost 80 per cent of their 999 older respondents used the best three points on a 7-point scale to indicate their QoL. Blane et al. (2002) reported a mean of 42.2 on a scale with a range 0–57 on the QoL measure they developed, again indicating some skewing towards the positive end of the scale with most study participants reporting reasonably good QoL. These typically skewed distributions of QoL ratings may partly reflect an editing process whereby people try to present themselves in a positive light.

In general, social desirability effects are stronger in face-to-face questioning as against more anonymous forms of testing (DeMaio 1984). Specific effects were found by Smith (1979) in that higher well-being was reported in face-to-face conditions as compared with surveys by postal means. However, in their GO programme study on transport and ageing, Gilhooly and her colleagues found no differences in QoL ratings using the 7-point Delighted–Terrible Faces rating scale when the data was collected via a postal questionnaire (Mean rating = 5.5, SD = 1.09, N = 1004) versus face-to-face interviews (Mean rating 5.5, SD = 1.06, N = 297).

Strack et al. (1990) found that self-presentation was affected by contextual effects. Higher well-being was reported in face-to-face interviews versus confidential self-report, except when the interviewer was obviously handicapped. This probably reflects a reluctance to stress how good one's life is to someone who is seen as less fortunate. However, if the handicapped person was present in the room as another participant filling in their own questionnaire, then subjective well-being reports were increased, presumably through a contrast effect. Comparing and contrasting one's QoL with other people is a common phenomenon, even if these other people are not present. In their GO transport study, M. Gilhooly and her colleagues (2002) found that when filling in the faces scale in interviews, older people frequently made comments in which they noted that their lives were better than many other older people. Beaumont et al. (2003) in their GO study on QoL of healthy older adults also noted that their study participants overwhelmingly adopted downward social comparison strategies when considering their QoL. In other words, those reporting higher QoL were more likely to see themselves as unlike those who were worse off. 'A lot of people here are a lot worse off than me' and '[You] gain a heightened awareness of all those who are in a worse position', were typical of the social comparison that participants made in Beaumont and Kenealy's (2003) study.

It appears then that to some degree self-reports of QoL may be edited and reported as somewhat higher than is privately felt. However, it may be noted that measures of how susceptible people are to social desirability effects in general are only weakly correlated (0.20) with well-being reports according to one study (Diener 1984). Overall, situational factors of the testing procedure may be more influential than individual differences.

Reconciling quantitative and qualitative asessments

As noted above, social desirability bias and other unknown mediating factors affect responses to questioning about perceived QoL. Likewise, it could be expected that qualitative and quantitative approaches might elicit very different answers to questions about the nature of QoL for older people. Bowling and her colleagues (2003) combined quantitative and qualitative approaches and, although the findings indicated considerable similarity in responses, there were some interesting differences.

Bowling et al. constructed a Quality of Life Survey Questionnaire which contained mainly structured questions and scales, but which also included open-ended questions placed at the beginning of the interview. The open-ended questions aimed to elicit descriptions of respondents' QoL, both good and bad, the respondents' priorities, and how QoL would be improved for themselves and for other people of their age. The open-ended questions were: 'First of all, thinking about your life as a whole, what is it that makes your life good – that is, the things that give your life quality? You may mention as many things as you like.' Respondents were asked next: 'And what is it that makes your life bad – that is the things that reduce the quality in your life? You may mention as many things as you like.' Respondents were asked which of all the areas of QoL they had mentioned was the single most important area to them: 'Thinking about all these good and bad things you have just mentioned which one is the most important to you?' (The interviewer prompted them first, 'You mentioned that . . .'.) This was followed with the question, 'And what single thing would improve the quality of your life?' Finally, respondents were asked, 'And what single thing, in your opinion, would improve the overall QoL for people of your age?' The open-ended questions on QoL were followed by a structured item asking people to rate the quality of their lives overall on a 7-point Likert category scale: 'So good it cannot be better', 'Very good', 'Good', 'Alright', 'Bad', 'Very bad', 'So bad it could not be worse'.

The open-ended questions were used as the opening ones in order to prevent respondent bias from the other, more specific questions and scales included the questionnaire. The use of the open-ended questions aimed to provide some insight into people's perceptions, without contamination from pre-fixed response codes and their format. This is a useful approach as it enables analysis of a large sample of respondents' own definitions and interpretations alongside standardized measurement scales and questions. It is more insightful than imposing structured, pre-defined response categories on people in relation to amorphous concepts such as QoL. It provides some evidence of the content validity for concepts and measures of QoL in older age, which necessitates questioning large numbers of representative older people, as well as supplementation of this method with qualitative research to provide richer insights into people's lives in order to provide contextual information on QoL.

The independent variables which were measured, in a structured format, in the wider survey, and which were derived from a literature review of QoL, included psychological self-construct: perceptions of self-efficacy (mastery and control), perceived risks of negative life events, optimism–pessimism bias, health values, physical functional status, health perceptions, psychological morbidity, personal social capital (perceived social network structure and support), and external social capital (local facilities, safety, problems within the area and neighbourliness of area), additional items on social networks, social comparisons and expectations, and standard socio-demographic and socio-economic characteristics and classifications.

Open responses were categorized into the following nine main ('root') themes: (1) social relationships; (2) social roles and activities; (3) health; (4) home and neighbourhood; (5) psychological well-being; (6) financial circumstances; (7) independence. The remaining two themes were 'society/ politics' and 'other'.

Gabriel and Bowling (2004) compared the results of an analytic regression model of theoretically derived indicators of self-evaluated overall QoL (closed survey items and scales) with the respondents' own definitions of QoL (categorization of open-ended survey questions), and with the views of a sub-sample of these respondents who were followed up in greater depth.

The main independent indicators of self-rated good QoL in the regression model, and which explained most of the variance in QoL ratings, were: making (downward) social comparisons between oneself and others and having positive social expectations of life; being optimistic; having better reported health and functional status; having more social activities; reported social support; less reported loneliness; better ratings of the quality of local facilities in their area of residence); and perceived safety of the area. The regression analysis model compared well overall with both of the empirically derived lay models based on the analysis of the open-ended survey responses and the in-depth follow-up interviews. The core components of QoL in older age, which were consistently emphasized by the three methods, were psychological variables (e.g. social expectations and comparisons, optimism–pessimism); health and functional status; and personal and external social capital.

The lay models, however, revealed the importance of the perception of having an adequate income, and of retaining independence and control over one's life. Comparing the findings of the quantitative and qualitative approaches, therefore, reveals the need to incorporate lay perceptions into a definition of broader QoL. As noted by Bowling and her colleagues, there is a need to move beyond the common emphasis on health and functional status, to a paradigm that includes self-constructs and cognitive mechanisms.

This study, which systematically combined qualitative and quantitative approaches to measurement, indicates that QoL is a multi-dimensional collection of objective and subjective areas of life, the parts of which can affect each other, as well as the sum. Because older people accommodate to deteriorating health, family, and social circumstances in order to feel good, individual coping mechanisms are of relevance to perceptions of QoL. Thus, and as noted earlier, personality characteristics such as optimism and self-mastery are of importance in managing the challenges of growing older. Definitions of QoL, as well as measurement, need, therefore, to include greater recognition of the dynamic interplay between perceptions, personal characteristics, circumstances, and surrounding social structures.

Conclusion

The GO Programme has not only raised awareness of the wide range of factors impacting on QoL in old age, but has contributed substantially to scholarly debate about the nature of the concept. This chapter extends that debate by examining several of the interesting issues associated with answering typical questions in QoL research. Recent research on the meaning and measurement of quality of life has shifted emphasis away from the previously negative paradigm of old age, with its focus on ill health, functional decline and poverty, towards a more positive view of old age as a natural component of the life span. Although limited resources, combined with ill health and the frailty of partners may restrict opportunities, for many old age is a period of life when one is freed from a number of structured social roles, for example, employment and the care of dependent children. The freedom to explore areas and activities which can provide personal fulfilment leads to new meanings for the term 'quality of life' in old age.

3

Dimensions of the inequalities in quality of life in older age

Paul Higgs, Martin Hyde, Sara Arber, David Blane, Elizabeth Breeze, James Nazroo and Dick Wiggins

Introduction

This chapter is concerned with examining the dimensions of the inequalities in quality of life (QoL) that exist among the older population of the United Kingdom. In particular, it will address how the bases and nature of inequalities have changed over time and how these have set up new challenges for those seeking to improve the lives of older people. The chapter will draw on four complementary studies conducted as part of the Growing Older programme: (1) analyses of a study of General Practitioner screening records of older people; (2) the General Household Survey; (3) the Fourth National Survey of Ethnic Minorities; and (4) a follow-up study of the Boyd-Orr Survey of 1936. In presenting findings from these studies, we hope to illustrate the importance of social factors, such as gender and ethnicity, for advancing understanding of inequalities in quality of later life at older ages.

Quality of life

The importance of QoL as a key issue for most industrialized societies is now generally accepted; however, what is less accepted is what actually constitutes it. Nations such as the UK have since the 1950s experienced growing economic prosperity, the eradication of most infectious diseases and increasing life expectancy. This has led some authors such as Inglehart (1997) to argue that we live in a 'post-materialist' culture where issues of QoL have replaced concerns of economic survival. The debates on the nature of life in what could be called 'post-scarcity societies' that feature in the work of Giddens (1994), Beck (1992) and Bauman (1999) reflect this position. Giddens suggests that what he calls the issues of life politics such as worries about the environment are more important to many than more established concerns such as poverty and inequality. In a similar, if not entwined, fashion Beck has argued that the 'risk society' is more concerned with the distribution of 'bads' rather than the distribution of 'goods'. Such a view is contentious in that it appears to sweep inequalities under the carpet, or at the least make them the outcome of individual agency (or lack of agency). Both these authors, implicitly, raise the question of whether QoL is therefore separate from the circumstances in which people find themselves. The obvious answer to this is that it is not. However it is important to recognize that the circumstances of post-materialist society may set up new contexts for understanding what constitutes QoL rather than merely subordinating it to non-materialist concerns. When we are addressing what is the nature of the inequalities in QoL evident in later life, we need to be aware that the idea of inequality needs to be extended to encompass more than simple lack.

Social participation is recognized as a major constituent part of QoL (Bowling 1995). However, the social forms in which people find themselves do not remain static but constantly change. This has been as true for later life as it has been for other parts of the lifecourse which have been affected by social changes such as the rise of consumerism, contraception and divorce. The present experience of later life is contextualized by retirement at younger ages as well as the expectation of a longer period of (healthy) post-working life more than was the case with previous cohorts. It is also the case that the people who are entering retirement are more similar to the rest of the population in terms of their experiences and motivations than may have been the case in the past (Hirsch 2000). This combination of factors suggests at the very least that QoL needs to be seen in terms of cohort or generation. As cohorts eventually die out, they are replaced by newer cohorts who have had different 'generational' experiences to those that had preceded them (Ryder 1985; Gilleard and Higgs 2002). While there has been considerable discussion about the existence of a 'welfare generation' that grew up and benefited from an expanding public sector (Hills 1995), less has been written about the effect of the 'sixties' generation entering retirement. The difference between the two generations and their expectations become more, rather than less, important once later life is reached. One such area is the interplay between generation and gender where the balance between autonomy and resources that emerges with the transformed domestic sphere has contradictory consequences. The importance of context, as we shall see, is also as important for those whose generational experiences were formed through the processes of migration. Inequalities in QoL, therefore, need to be related to the changing environments in which later life is being lived.

That QoL is not assessed in these terms is apparent from the way that it is traditionally studied. Generally, QoL is reduced to proxies or to individualized scales (Hyde et al. 2003). In particular, QoL in older populations is often reduced to health or social contact. Bowling (1997) points out that it is no longer possible to measure QoL simply as a medical outcome. However, using other simple proxies such as income get us little further, particularly when we are trying to understand the unequal structuring of QoL. Instead, we need to examine how the various social structures such as class, gender and ethnicity interplay to enable (or restrict) older people to engage with the opportunities available to them in general. In the same way that it is no longer acceptable to see health-related QoL only in terms of survival or cure, this can apply to QoL more generally. In other words, QoL needs to be seen as an expanding concept rather than a restricted one. In contemporary society that may mean a focus on leisure pursuits (Midwinter 1992; Scase and Scales 2000) and foreign travel (Burnett 1991). That these activities may seem frivolous does not detract from their significance, but rather indicates the new sites for inequality.

Socio-economic disadvantage and poor quality of life among older people

A major context of QoL is the socio-economic circumstances in which people find themselves. However, the question that emerges both from research and from our concern with QoL, is, how do these circumstances influence QoL? While the relations between poor socio-economic circumstances and both poor physical and mental health are well established, relatively little is known about how different aspects of socio-economic status (SES) act on health. This becomes more complex when data from a working population have shown that different measures of SES have different effects on self-reported health (Singh-Manoux et al. 2002). Consequently, when looking at a post-working population, the different aspects that constitute SES might be more or less important. For example, housing tenure is correlated with material resources but in old age owner-occupation does not necessarily mean high income or good housing conditions (Department of Environment 1998). It does, however, convey other, non-material, benefits such as status and pride (Macintyre et al. 2000) as home ownership was rarer in older generations than now. These older generations established their careers when jobs were highly hierarchical in respect to income and status and the work environment was often hazardous. Consequently, social class could influence health through a combination of experiences, income available, and psychosocial factors influenced by degree of control over life. One of the projects in the Growing Older programme addressed these issues by using secondary data analysis to assess whether poor QoL, defined in terms of standard instruments for morale and health-related functioning, varied systematically by socio-economic status.

The study

The data in the study used came from the Medical Research Council (MRC) trial of the assessment and management of older people in the community. This study focused on methods of administration and follow-up for the annual health checks that family doctors were contracted to provide for all people aged 75 years and over. The General Practice was the unit of randomization and the trial's design and methods are described elsewhere (Fletcher et al. 2002). Baseline information about SES and housing tenure was gained from QoL interviews undertaken in a randomly selected subset of 23 practices of the 106 practices recruited. Some 8707 of the 9547 people from the 23 practices eligible to participate in the trial were interviewed at baseline. However, 2249 (26 per cent) were in excluded tenure categories. After further exclusions for missing information 5987 (69 per cent) of responders were included in the analysis. Although response to the QoL interview varied little by gender and age, more women and older respondents were in the excluded tenures (25 per cent of men and 48 per cent of women aged at least 85 years compared to 13 per cent and 22 per cent who were aged under 80 years). The included group had lower prevalence of poor QoL than the excluded group, for example, 13 per cent of the analysis sample had poor home management and 19 per cent poor morale compared to 34 per cent and 25 per cent respectively of those excluded.

Quality of life

Trained interviewers, independent of the practice, administered the interviews in the privacy of patients' homes. The core questionnaire included four dimensions from the UK version of the Sickness Impact Profile (SIP) (Bergner et al. 1981) and the Philadelphia Geriatric Morale Scale (Lawton 1975), a

17-item measure of morale developed for use with older people. SIP specifies limitations and in this study had three response options: 'no', 'yes and due to health' and 'yes and not due to health'. Both forms of yes were combined for these analyses. The four dimensions were home management (for example, shopping, housework), mobility at home and outside, self-care ranging from being bed-bound to limited dexterity, and social interaction including frequency and emotional aspects of contact. Housing tenure was included as an indicator of SES in post-working life and social class, representing SES achieved during working life. Data on current residence and main occupation in working life and that of male spouse was collected in the interview. The analysis refers to people who were living alone or with their spouse because it was judged that housing tenure most clearly reflected socio-economic position for this subset. No clear socio-economic status is attached to sheltered housing and residential homes and people's housing tenure may not reflect the personal material resources and status of those living with other than spouse. Main lifetime occupation was collected and social class was coded manually using the 1991 classification of occupations (OPCS 1991). Women who were ever married were assigned their (former) husband's social class where possible.

Results

For all the measures used there is a very similar pattern with those in the most disadvantaged situation more likely to report poor health, poor functioning and low morale. Compared to the reference group, all other groups had an increased likelihood of reporting problems with home management (HM) and mobility (MOB). Those in the most disadvantaged group, in social class IV or V living in the social sector, are over twice as likely to report a mobility problem as those from social class I or II who own their property. The likelihood of reporting a problem increases as one moves down the social classes and is higher for those who live in the social sector within each of the classes. Compared to the reference group, all other groups have an increased risk of reporting problems with self-care (SC). As with mobility problems, there is a clear evidence of a gradient by social class, with those in social classes IV or V who own their own residence nearly twice as likely to report these problems. There is also clear evidence of the additive effect of living in the social sector. For all social classes, save those in classes IV or V, those who live in the social sector have a considerably higher risk than their owner-occupier counterparts. For social interaction (SI), all but those from social classes I or II who have 'other' residential arrangements have an increased likelihood of

31

reporting poor social interaction. There is clear evidence of the effects of both social class, with those in the lowest social classes having the highest risk of reporting poor interaction, and of living in the social sector. However the additive effects of residential status do not follow the social class gradient but attenuate class differences considerably. The results for morale show a similar pattern although there is a diminution of the odds ratio for those in the lowest social classes in both residential statuses.

As poor functioning was unlikely to have existed prior to retirement, we can be confident that social class preceded poor functioning, and we reduced the scope for distortion from reverse causation between housing tenure and QoL by confining analysis to people living alone or with spouse. Nearly a quarter of those in social classes IV/V were living in excluded tenures compared to under one in ten of those in social classes I/II, so there was probably an underestimation of the extent of socio-economic variation. Although other health or behavioural factors may explain the socio-economic differences, they could be part of the pathway between socio-economic status and limited functioning. The cumulative effects of social class (acquired many years earlier), and current housing tenure suggest that older people do not escape the legacy of their individual socio-economic history and are not immune from current socio-economic influences. The action needed to reduce those differentials may differ in whole or part from action appropriate for younger groups, for example, multiple morbidities may already exist and therefore treatment may be a bigger consideration for them than it is for younger age groups. Improving the welfare of older people, a stated objective of government policy, involves efforts to reduce health inequalities among this population.

The effects of gender and marital status on quality of material life in older age

Another important context for QoL is the question of how gender and marital status connect with material inequalities. Literature on inequalities in later life usually focuses on gender and social class, and sometimes, also race/ethnicity without necessarily looking at how these factors interact (Arber and Ginn 1991). However, feminist writers have stressed the importance of analysing the interaction between class, race and gender (Calasanti and Slevin 2001). In particular, marital status is an example of gendered power relations that differentiate both men and women across their lifecourse and have an effect on QoL.

A lot is already known about the effects of marital status on health and mortality for both men and women (Welin et al. 1985; Lillard and Waite 1995). However there has been little research that has looked at how these dynamics might affect QoL in older ages.

Older women's and men's current financial circumstances are intimately tied to their previous role in the labour market and thus their pension acquisition. The gendered organization of caring for children and partners means that older married, widowed and divorced women's employment careers will have been constrained by caring responsibilities (Ginn 2003). The marital status distribution of the older population is rapidly changing, with profound implications for future generations of older people (Arber et al. 2003b; Arber and Ginn 2004). Widowhood is normative for older women, since half of women over the age of 65 in Britain are widowed. The common experience of widowhood for women contrasts with the norm for men, that they remain married until their death. However, this may blinker us to issues that the minority of older widowed men face, as well as the small but growing proportions who are divorced.

The study

The study used pooled cross-sectional data from five waves of the General Household Survey (GHS) 1993–1996 and 1998 (no GHS was conducted in 1997). This produced a sample of over 15,000 men and women aged over 65 years. Logistic regression models are used to compare the effects of marital status on economic circumstances for older women and men. Four categories of marital status, married/cohabiting, widowed, divorced/separated and never married, were created for both men and women yielding eight groups. Age, banded in five-year groups, was controlled for in all analyses.

Three dichotomous indicators of quality of material life are examined: low household income, renting (rather than owning) a home, and not having a car within the household. Low household income is measured as being in the lowest quartile (25 per cent) of the income distribution of those over 65.[1] For all the analyses, married men are defined as the reference category, thus any group with an odds ratio higher than 1.00 has a greater likelihood of disadvantage compared to married men.

Results

Figure 3.1a shows that divorced women are the group most likely to have low household income in later life with an odds ratio 4.7 times higher than married

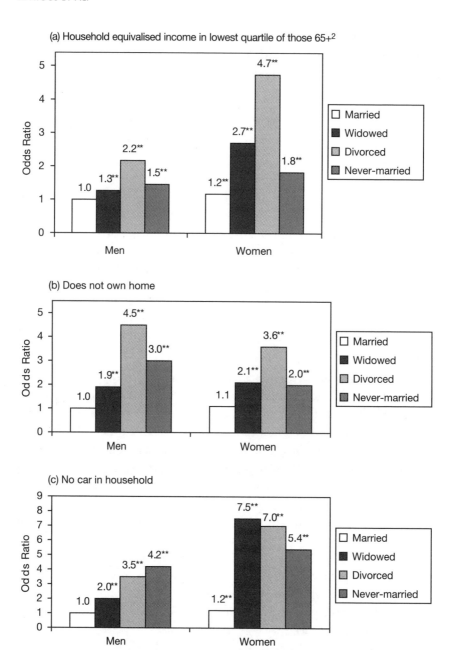

Figure 3.1 Material circumstances by gender and marital status, odds ratios[1], age 65+[2]

men. Widows are the next most financially disadvantaged, with an odds ratio 2.7 times higher than for married men. The household income of widowers is not very different from that of married men, thus among men (unlike women) little financial penalty is attached to widowhood. Divorced men are the most financially disadvantaged among older men, but their income is much higher than divorced women. There are much greater income differences among older women by marital status, than among older men.

Other aspects of quality of material life include home and car ownership. Home ownership represents an important capital asset, with married men and women the most advantaged, and divorced men and women the most disadvantaged (Figure 3.1b). Divorced older men have even higher odds of renting than divorced women. Men who have never married have much higher odds of renting (OR = 3.0) than married men, and higher than women who have never married. Older widows and widowers have about twice the odds of renting compared to married men and women, suggesting that renting is associated with widowhood *per se*, since there are no clear differences by gender.

For both men and women, having a car is important for maintaining independence – the ability to shop, visit, enjoy leisure facilities, help with grandchildren, attend hospital appointments, and so on. Among older cohorts of women the norm was to depend on their husband for transport, with fewer holding driving licences themselves. Thus, for women, widowhood or divorce may represent more than the loss of a breadwinner and partner – it may include the loss of mobility. Car ownership varies fundamentally by gender – all groups of older women without a partner are disadvantaged compared with men and married women. Although we can expect the gender division of car ownership to lessen for future cohorts in later life, older women may still lack the financial resources to run a car (Ginn 2003).

Across these three measures of material inequality, being married is associated with material well-being for both women and men, but this advantaged state is the province of nearly three-quarters of older men and only two-fifths of women. Widowed and divorced women in these cohorts are disadvantaged, having often spent much of their lifecourse subjugating their own occupational career to their role as wife and mother. Divorced older men and women are particularly disadvantaged groups – these groups are projected to grow substantially in the future, reflecting cohort changes in divorce rates in Britain (Arber and Ginn 2004). Despite the fact that many never-married older women were well-educated 'career women', their income and car ownership levels are lower than those of never-married men. To understand the financial and material well-being of older people, it is necessary to consider the 'interaction' of gender *and* marital status, since there are different gender-related processes impacting on women and men according to marital status, reflecting their lifecourse engagement in paid work and family building. Gender differences by marital status largely reflect gender relations across the lifecourse; ever-partnered women's caring responsibilities have constrained their employment participation, while men without partners have not benefited from the support provided by wives for their employment careers. What this research points to is the importance of both individual lives and the patterning of social processes in creating the contexts for QoL. The fact that the more recently retired come from cohorts with higher divorce rates also points to the importance of social change in creating the conditions for later life.

Ethnic inequalities in quality of life at older ages

The QoL of older ethnic minorities living in the UK has received relatively little attention compared to more established inequalities such as those based on material circumstances or gender. One obvious reason is the low numbers of older people from ethnic minorities. Only 3.5 per cent of the male population aged over 50 years and less than 2.5 per cent of the female population aged over 50 years were from non-white backgrounds (Gjonça and Calderwood 2003). There is, however, a pressing need to understand the conditions and dynamics of ageing which members of ethnic minorities face in later life. Migration and consequent employment and health histories, formation of migrant communities and disruption of family networks, are all important factors unique to these cohorts. The study reported here revealed six factors that influenced the QoL of older people from ethnic minorities: (1) having a role; (2) support networks; (3) income and wealth; (4) health; (5) having time; and (6) independence.

The study

A mixture of qualitative and quantitative techniques was used to explore the distribution of factors that might affect QoL across four ethnic groups (Caribbean, Indian, Pakistani and white) and to examine how these were differentially experienced and valued across the various groups. Quantitative data was taken from the Fourth National Survey of Ethnic Minorities (Modood et al. 1997; Bajekal et al. 2004). This study was also used as the sample frame from which to draw a purposive sample for the qualitative element covering

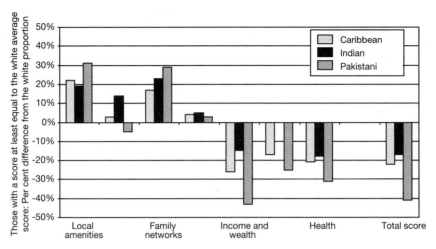

Figure 3.2 Ethnic differences in factors contributing to quality of life at older ages

men and women, different ages (within a broad range of 60–74), different class groups and different regions. The qualitative work focused on ethnic differences in influences on and levels of QoL (Grewal et al. 2004). A total of 73 in-depth qualitative interviews were carried out, covering broad pre-determined topics and additional, unanticipated, topics raised by respondents themselves. Figure 3.2 summarizes descriptive findings from the quantitative analysis of the circumstances of older ethnic minority people from three illustrative groups (Caribbean, Indian and Pakistani) in comparison with white people. It covers dimensions of the local environment, social participation and networks, material circumstances and health. Scores above zero indicate a favourable situation in comparison with the white group, while those below zero indicate a disadvantaged situation. The total score sums the various dimensions shown in the figure to give an overall comparison, one that suggests that older ethnic minority people fare considerably worse than their white counterparts. However, this pattern is not consistent across the individual dimensions represented in the figure. Below we describe these findings in the context of the qualitative data.

Material conditions

Of all the factors demonstrated in Figure 3.2, the gap between older people in the white and ethnic minority groups was largest for income and wealth, as well as for housing conditions. These findings were reinforced by the qualitative interviews. These suggested that income and wealth were affected by occupational histories and, consequently, varied across both ethnic and gender groups. Women in all groups tended to be located among those receiving a state pension only, because their patterns of work had meant that they had not contributed sufficiently to a pension scheme. This was also the case for ethnic minority men, typically because of long-term sickness, or unemployment prior to retirement, which had affected their pension contributions.

Health

The pattern of differences in health shown in Figure 3.2 is also large and clear, with significant variations between groups by ethnicity. All the ethnic minority groups had significantly poorer health scores compared with the white group; and of the three minority groups, Pakistani people had significantly poorer health. The qualitative interviews suggested that Pakistani men suffered especially poor health because of their former employment. However, perceptions varied on what constituted good health. The continuation of mental health was valued over physical health.

Quality of neighbourhood

On average, respondents in all three ethnic minority groups rated the availability of amenities in their local neighbourhood as significantly better than respondents in the white group did. However, the ratings of the quality of the local area in terms of crime and environment did not show a clear difference between white and non-white groups. This is in direct contrast to estimates of the relative deprivation of areas where people live, as, for example, measured by the Index of Deprivation 2000. This shows that those wards where white people live are, on average, less deprived than those where ethnic minority people live and that among ethnic minorities Pakistani people live in the most deprived wards and have the poorest access to service. The qualitative findings suggest that the 'mismatch' between respondents' assessment of their neighbourhoods and the formal assessments may be a consequence of ethnic minority people either specifically settling in areas that had, for example, an appropriate place of worship, shops or clubs, or alternatively investing in developing the local infrastructure to meet their needs.

Support networks

The qualitative interviews identified support as a key contributor of quality to an individual's life. Partner, family, friends, and religion emerged as the main sources of support. These interviews suggested that for ethnic minority people migration had had a disruptive effect on both family and friendship networks. The consequent reduction of social networks, for example, loss of friendships formed from schooldays or during the transition into work, may explain their higher level of association with family, illustrated by their scores on contact with family shown in Figure 3.2, which were significantly higher for older people in the Indian and Pakistani groups compared to the white group. The interviews also revealed religion as a significant provider of emotional support for respondents in all ethnic groups, especially in times of grief and pain. Religious organizations were also a source of practical support for ethnic minority people, for example, funding trips to their country of origin, or providing domestic help for housebound older people.

Having time and having a role

The qualitative interviews showed that either as a result of retirement or of children growing up, respondents found that they had more free time as they got older. People in good health who had a certain level of income welcomed this freedom to travel, pursue hobbies and take a more active role in religion. A more unwelcome aspect of retirement or children growing up was the loss of a sense of purpose or role that it sometimes entailed. Family, community, religion and voluntary or paid work were the main providers of a social role. For white English older people, voluntary work was likely to be undertaken through local or national charities, while for ethnic minority older people it tended to be channelled through the local and ethnically/religious specific community. In other words, participation in the community was equally popular across ethnic groups, but the sources that provided that role varied between minority and majority groups.

Summary of findings

In summary, while indicating important dimensions of inequality, this brief description of the position of older ethnic minority people indicates that the situation is a little more complex than is suggested by claims that older ethnic minority people simply face multiple sources of disadvantage. The quantitative part of the study revealed extensive differences across ethnic groups in most of the established influences on QoL that were covered in the data. Factors that are typically included in research concerned with inequality (material conditions, health, crime and physical environment and formal assessments of social participation) revealed a familiar pattern. The white group tended to have the best scores. However, for those influences concerned with less formal elements of the community, social support and perceptions of the quality of local amenities, the differences were reversed.

Lifecourse and present-day influences on quality of life in older age

As has already been mentioned, the circumstances and hence the QoL in old age cannot be separated from the experience of ageing. The concept of the lifecourse has become increasingly popular area of research in both social gerontology (Dannefer 2003) and health sciences (Blane et al. 1997; Kuh and Ben-Shlomo 1997; Blane, 1999; Graham, 2002). Epidemiological studies have demonstrated lifecourse influences on both physical (Montgomery et al. 2000) and mental health (Power et al. 2002) in later life. However, little work has been done to look at the lifecourse influences on QoL in early old age. The fourth and final study concerned with inequalities in QoL in older age combined a range of lifecourse and contemporary data about people's circumstances with a novel measure of QoL.

Quality of life

A new measure of QoL was developed in response to the widely acknowledged lack of theory in the area. Many existing scales are not explicit about the theoretical model and, thus, the concept that was being measured (Gill and Feinstein 1994). The main problems were, either that proxy measures such as health, financial status or social networks were used to measure QoL, or that QoL was regarded as a completely subjective phenomenon. The measure of QoL was based on the theory of needs satisfaction. The items were tested with focus groups, cognitive interviews and by statistical analyses. These produced a 19-item scale labelled the CASP-19 (Higgs et al. 2003; Hyde et al 2003).

The study

The respondents in this study were drawn from a unique sample. As children, they were surveyed between 1937 and 1939 by a team of medical and nutritional scientists under the direction of Sir John Boyd Orr. Almost all of these records were retrieved in 1996 and, using the National Health Service Central Register, the Office of National Statistics was able to successfully trace 85 per cent of the children who participated in the original study. Following the retrieval of these records, a stratified random sample was drawn from the full

Boyd Orr cohort. In 1997–98 retrospective data were collected, using the life-grid method (Berney and Blane 1997), from 296 members of this stratified random sample. Full household, residential and occupational histories were recorded; and physiological and anthropometric measurements were made. These sample members proved broadly representative of their age peers within the British population (Blane et al. 1999). In 2000 these individuals were mailed a self-completion questionnaire about their QoL.

Distribution of quality of life in early old age

The distribution of the scores for the whole sample shows that there is a range of QoL in early old age. Men have a slightly higher QoL than do women. Similarly, there was little difference between the QoL of those from non-manual occupations as compared to those from manual occupations. There was a pronounced difference in the QoL of the younger and older members of the sample. The 'young-old', those people aged under 70, had a much higher QoL than the 'older-old', those over 70.

Lifecourse effects on quality of life

The accumulation of disadvantage over the lifecourse at home and at work had a negative effect on later QoL (Blane et al. 2004). There was evidence also that early retirement among the socio-economically disadvantaged was associated subsequently with reduced QoL; a relationship which was not found among their more socially advantaged peers. The most important single life event that had an effect on QoL in older age was purchasing one's own home (notably when social housing was sold off) (Blane et al. 2004). However, as Table 3.1 shows, when the effects of exposure to disadvantage across the lifecourse influence were examined together with present-day factors, the latter were shown to exert the most powerful effect on QoL in later life.

The effects of health and wealth on quality of life

There were significant differences in the QoL between those who had a limiting long-standing illness and those who did not. Owner-occupiers had a higher QoL than those who continued to rent their property. There was, however, no relationship between the number of state or occupational pensions that the household received and the individual's QoL. By combining measures of health and wealth we created groups to test the relative effect of health and wealth on QoL. Four groups were created: (1) those with good health and good wealth; (2) those with good health and poor wealth; (3) those with poor health and

Table 3.1 Cumulative effects of social class and housing tenure in old age among those still independent in old age. Risk ratios (95% CI) for poor quality of life

QOL[1]	Current housing tenure	Social class [2]			
		I/II	IIINM	IIIM	IV/V
HM	Owner-occupier	1.00	1.12 (0.9, 1.4)	1.63 (1.4, 1.9)	1.47 (1.2, 1.9)
	Social sector	1.28 (1.0, 1.6)	1.43 (1.0, 2.1)	2.09 (1.6, 2.8)	1.89 (1.4, 2.5)
	Other	1.23 (1.0, 1.5)	1.38 (1.0, 2.0)	2.00 (1.5, 2.7)	1.81 (1.3, 2.6)
MOB	Owner-occupier	1.00	1.12 (0.9, 1.4)	1.62 (1.4, 1.9)	1.71 (1.4, 2.1)
	Social sector	1.31 (1.1, 1.6)	1.47 (1.0, 2.1)	2.12 (1.6, 2.8)	2.23 (1.7, 2.9)
	Other	1.16 (0.9, 1.4)	1.30 (0.9, 1.9)	1.88 (1.4, 2.6)	1.98 (1.4, 2.7)
SC[3]	Owner-occupier	1.00	1.17 (1.0, 1.4)	1.46 (1.2, 1.8)	1.85 (1.5, 2.3)
	Social sector	1.97 (1.4, 2.8)	1.93 (1.2, 3.0)	2.31 (1.9, 2.9)	1.77 (1.4, 2.3)
	Other	1.38 (0.9, 2.1)	1.54 (0.9, 2.6)	2.20 (1.5, 3.2)	1.38 (0.8, 2.4)
SI[3]	Owner-occupier	1.00	1.23 (0.9, 1.7)	1.53 (1.2, 1.9)	1.86 (1.5, 2.3)
	Social sector	2.29 (1.7, 3.0)	2.04 (1.4, 3.0)	2.33 (1.8, 3.1)	2.06 (1.5, 2.8)
	Other	0.73 (0.4, 1.2)	1.48 (0.7, 3.3)	1.86 (1.3, 2.7)	1.63 (1.0, 2.7)
Morale	Owner-occupier	1.00	1.28 (1.1, 1.5)	1.45 (1.2, 1.7)	1.31 (1.1, 1.6)
	Social sector	1.33 (1.1, 1.6)	1.71 (1.4, 2.2)	1.94 (1.6, 2.3)	1.74 (1.5, 2.0)
	Other	1.21 (1.0, 1.5)	1.55 (1.2, 2.1)	1.75 (1.4, 2.2)	1.58 (1.2, 2.0)

Numbers (%) of
analysis sample

	All				
Owner-occupier	4291 (71.7)	1923 (32.1)	583 (9.7)	1327 (22.2)	458 (7.7)
Social sector	1223	100 (1.7)	112	608 (10.2)	403 (6.7)

Notes: [1] Odds ratios after controlling for five year age groups (65–9, 70–4, 75–9, 80–4, 85+); reference category is married men with odds defined as 1.00.

[2] Household income having adjusted for household composition using the McClements Scale.

[3] Base Numbers: Men – Married – 4673, Widowed – 1196, Divorced/separated – 284, Never married – 389; Women – Married – 3651, Widowed – 4160, Divorced/separated – 372, Never married – 596. Significance of difference from the reference category, *$p < 0.05$, **$p < 0.01$.

Source: General Household Survey 1993–96, 1998.

good wealth; and, finally, (4) those with poor health and poor wealth. The general pattern was that those with good health and good wealth had the best QoL, followed by those with good health and poor wealth while those with poor health and poor wealth suffered the worst QoL. These results indicate that health is more important than wealth for the QoL of this cohort.

The effects of social networks and local area on quality of life in early old age

Three components of social networks were measured: (1) quality of contact; (2) frequency of contact; and (3) density of contact. The majority of the sample reported good quality of social contact, seeing some at least once a week and having one or two close friends. Both the quality of social contact and the density of social contact had a significant, positive, effect on QoL. Frequency of contact, on the other hand, did not have a significant effect on QoL. Perceptions of local area had a weak effect on QoL (Wiggins et al. 2004).

Despite the lack of a significant effect of the lifecourse measures used in this study on the QoL of the respondents, the lifecourse forms an essential component for our understanding of old age. The ability of people to enjoy a good QoL is likely to be dependent on their ability to accumulate human and financial capital throughout their life. Thus, it is probable that the lifecourse acts in an indirect manner on QoL by influencing those contemporary factors which, in turn, affect QoL. However, such a distinction masks an implicit lifecourse element inherent in all contemporary factors. For example, pension entitlements are dependent on working histories, social networks are established over time and individual health, especially in terms of chronic illness, is acquired over life.

Discussion

The research findings reported above demonstrate the existence of very real inequalities in later life; they also draw our attention to the fact that such inequalities are complex in both origin and effect. Acknowledging the existence of inequalities in the many forms that they take, however, is not sufficient to locate their effect on QoL. What *have* been identified in these studies are possible influences on QoL. Such influences need to be separated from QoL *per se* if we are not to make the mistake of reducing it to one dimension of life such as health or wealth. Instead, as was outlined at the beginning of the chapter, QoL is contextualized by the social environment in which people experience life and conditioned by the social processes that individuals have lived through.

To understand the context of inequalities in QoL in the period when the research was being carried out, we have to know something about the average experiences of retired people in the UK at the time. While calculations of income are fraught with difficulty in terms of comparability and meaningfulness, it is difficult to dispute that the income levels of the retired population have been improving over the period when these studies were being conducted. This is true for both average income and for position in the overall distribution of income (Department of Work and Pensions (2003), Pensioners' income series 2001/2). The paradox is that this improvement has been accompanied by a growing inequality within the older population as the retired started to reflect the inequalities of the wider society rather than be over-representative of poverty. This transformation has, as we have seen, affected some more than others. Pointing this out and drawing out its causation are important for research, but this is not necessarily the same as describing its impact on QoL. As the CASP-19 project, looking at a relatively young sample of retired people, demonstrated QoL scores were not dramatically affected by income. This is not so surprising in a population where participation in a culture not defined by poverty and lack is possible for most. Drawing on the results presented in this chapter, it is true that the situation for some older members of ethnic minorities, and for some older women, does indicate that their lives are deeply affected by inequalities and a lack of resources (Table 3.2). However, for even for those most disadvantaged by low income and disability, the provision of extra income is not just about the alleviation of lack. It can be seen as a way of experiencing some of the components of a more generally accepted QoL. In a paper examining citizenship and social exclusion of older people, Craig (2004) points out that the importance of increased benefit income for many disabled older people lay not in meeting financial hardship as such, but in the independence and choice that it gave them. In particular, extra income allowed them to participate in their communities and maintain their personal identities. This included being able to buy presents or travelling to visit family overseas. Consequently, it is important to address the issue of what inequalities in resources practically mean in the context of people's lives rather than just impute them from harder data such as income or health. As the research projects show, while these have an impact, they are not the same as QoL.

If QoL has to be contextualized by reference to expectations and inequalities by what constraints are placed in the way of full social participation, then

Table 3.2 Summary of regression analyses for CASP-19 as the dependent variable

Term	Base	+Hazard	+Legacy	+Social capital	+Social network	+Recent life events
Constant	43.05	44.62	50.50	47.15	39.21	39.81
Female		−0.33	−0.36	−0.28	−0.25	−1.59	−1.62*
Over 70	−4.25	−4.40	−3.87	−3.63	−3.37	−2.98
Lifecourse Hazards		−0.07	−0.04	−0.02	−0.03	0.01
Non-owner			−0.95	−0.82*	−1.04	−1.11
Retirement (no choice)			−0.77	−1.08	−1.73	−0.99
Poor pension			−4.90	−4.38	−4.16	−3.86
Poor health			−2.23*	−1.97*	−2.08	−1.88*
No car			0.47	0.04	−0.61	−0.56
Misery				0.31	−0.08	−0.04
Community				0.66	0.22	0.05
Deprived				−3.98	−2.95	−2.45
Affluence				0.05	−0.22	0.05
Density					0.57	0.57
Quality					0.49	0.46
Frequency					0.01	−0.01
Recent life event						−5.44
R-square	0.05	0.08	0.17	0.23	0.35	0.40
Change in R-square		0.03	0.09	0.06	0.12	0.05

Note: Regression Coefficients are emboldened whenever $p < 0.05$ across all replicate analyses. An asterisk (*) denotes that a coefficient approaches conventional significance ($p < 0.10$).

these expectations are conditioned by social processes that affect individual life-courses. This can be easily seen in the situations of women and members of migrant minority ethnic groups. Their lives have often been over-determined by the social processes surrounding gender and the domestic economy, on the one hand, or those surrounding racialization, on the other, or maybe both. The effects of these conditioning processes can be seen in the inequalities outlined earlier. When we are looking for the effects of social class, these effects are seen less clearly. Certainly, housing tenure would seem to be a consequence of social class membership, but since the 1980s council housing has been affected by deliberate social policies designed to marginalize those occupying such housing. The effects of such policies, it could be suggested, were to increase the negative consequences of 'ageing in place', with those with the means taking flight to better locations or transforming their environments through buying their council houses. The changing nature of housing tenure and occupational structure are just two (albeit highly salient) conditioning processes for understanding the impact of inequalities on QoL through the lifecourses of individuals.

However, it would be incorrect to conclude that the lifecourse is overwhelmingly the determinant conditioning process in understanding inequalities in QoL. When present-day and lifecourse influences were examined together, the former exerted a much more powerful effect on QoL in later life than did lifecourse factors (Wiggins et al. 2004). Indeed, decisions such as choosing to buy a council house had a positive effect on CASP-19 scores suggesting that QoL can be improved by actions unrelated to lifecourse disadvantage.[2] Addressing the social context of QoL brings us back to the beginning of this chapter, where we questioned the nature of QoL. In contemporary Britain, this has to be seen in relation to participation in a society of relative affluence, in which consumption and leisure are major aspirations. That these are increasingly generational aspirations needs to be accepted. The retirement of the baby boomer generation is both a context and a conditioning process (Gilleard and Higgs 2002); their experiences will define what constitutes good QoL as well as how evenly it is distributed. It is in this light that inequalities and their effects will be evaluated and not purely in terms of an external proxy for QoL.

Conclusion

This chapter has been concerned with inequalities in QoL among older people. It has sought to show that demonstrating inequalities in resources or health is not simply the same as demonstrating inequalities in QoL. While such inequalities have the capacity to influence QoL, the processes by which they do so are complex and not easily disentangled. We have shown that the significance of inequalities for understanding QoL lies in their impact in restricting social participation as well as being deficits of income and health. Quality of life also needs to be seen as being situated in particular contexts and conditioned by changing social circumstances that set the parameters for social participation. In such circumstances, the important inequalities are those that restrict access to good quality life rather than being sufficient 'reified' realities of their own. As important as the task of delineating the forms taken by inequalities is the task of finding out what their consequences are, and how they affect individual QoL. In utilizing the studies we have drawn upon, we hope that we have demonstrated some of these, but we are aware that there are plenty more needing investigation and attention.

Acknowledgements

The authors would like to acknowledge the hard work done by the many researchers on the four projects reported here; Kate Davidson, Kim Perren, Debora Price, Ini Grewal, Madhavi Bajekal, Jane Lewis, Saffron Karlson, Astrid Fletcher, Paul Wilkinson, Dee Jones, Amina Latif, and Chris Bulpitt. We would also like to thank all of the respondents of all the projects for their cooperation.

Notes

1 Income levels were adjusted to 1998 values using the Retail Price Index, and household composition is adjusted using McClements income equivalising scales (Department of Work and Pensions 2002).

2 Of course, earlier influences shape QoL by shaping present-day influences, but are these earlier influences as powerful now in determining QoL as they might once of been? It is at least arguable that some of the features of consumer culture are more amenable to mass participation than the more austere social conditions that marked post-working lives in the 1960s and 1970s.

4

Getting out and about

Caroline Holland, Leonie Kellaher, Sheila Peace,
Thomas Scharf, Elizabeth Breeze, Jane Gow and
Mary Gilhooly

It's very important [to get out]; otherwise you can vegetate, become inward looking.
(Respondent, Study Four)

I can't go on my own because I can't walk . . . I mustn't go out without an escort
from here. That is another thing you mustn't do from here [residential care
home]. (Woman aged 85, Study One)

Introduction

People in general want and need to get out and about. Older people are no
exception: shopping, working, socializing, using services, and giving and
receiving support. Beyond the practical, most older people also relish the
pleasures and challenges of life beyond the home and strive to maintain for as
long as possible their independence and ability to get out and about. If this
becomes difficult, people tend to find ways indoors to ring the changes and
remain connected with the world outside. In this chapter we will present
evidence of how older people can be highly strategic in making decisions
about and interacting with the several layers of 'environment' within our four
Growing Older programme studies. Importantly, we consider the significance
of venturing beyond the 'home range' by public or private transport and
the effects on morale of being able to get out and about. We suggest that the
capacity to make and execute choices in moving around within and outside
the home is crucial, and not simply to accomplish the necessary and desirable
activities of daily living. It is essential to a person's sense of who they are
and how they are situated in their material and social worlds, and, as a
consequence, to their quality of life (QoL).

Four projects

This chapter is based on findings from four projects which varied methodologically from large-scale and highly quantitative to multi-method and qualitative studies of small samples in specific geographical locations. The discussion sections that follow are based on points of commonality which emerged from the separate analyses by the project teams of their own data. The four projects are as follows.

Study One: *Environment and Identity in Later Life: A Cross-Setting Study* (Peace et al. 2003). This study involved ten focus groups followed by case studies with older people living in a wide range of types of accommodation from residential care homes to detached houses, and in settlements from small villages to a London borough. From group discussions of issues related to living environments and sense of identity, a series of questionnaire schedules and an interview tool were devised and used in more in-depth discussions with 54 individuals in Bedford, Northamptonshire, and the London borough of Haringey.

Study Two: *Older People in Deprived Neighbourhoods: Social Exclusion and Quality of Life in Old Age* (Scharf et al. 2003). This study entailed face-to-face interviews with 600 people aged 60 and over in nine electoral wards of Liverpool, Manchester, and the London borough of Newham. These were the three English local authorities that ranked lowest (worst) in the 1998 Index of Local Deprivation (DETR 1998). This phase was followed by 130 in-depth interviews in the same areas, including interviews with older people from a range of minority ethnic groups.

Study Three: *Inequalities in Quality of Life Among People Aged 75 Years and Over in Great Britain* (Breeze et al. 2002). This study surveyed 8000 people aged 75 years and over registered with 23 general practices that were taking part in an MRC Trial of the assessment and management of older people in the community. Quality of life was assessed at baseline and at a 36-month follow-up, measured by the Philadelphia Geriatric Center Morale Scale and four sets of questions from the Functional Limitations Profile (FLP), including mobility.

Study Four: *Transport and Ageing: Extending Quality of Life via Public and Private Transport* (Gilhooly et al. 2003). This was a multi-method study conducted in Paisley, rural Renfrewshire, and inner and outer London, which examined the views of people aged 45 and over. It involved 17 focus groups, street surveys, a postal survey of people aged 18 and over drawn from electoral rolls (1128 returns), and 306 interviews with a stratified quota sample of older people. Interviews were also conducted with transport providers and other stakeholders.

Further summary details of these four projects are published as Growing Older Findings (http://www.shef.ac.uk/uni/projects/gop/) and we wish to acknowledge here the generous contribution of all those older people and others who took part in our projects. In the following discussion the projects will, for brevity, be referred to as Studies One to Four.

In its broadest sense, the term 'environment' encompasses the micro-environments that constitute the home, through to macro meanings of the urban and the rural. Rather than treating 'environment' simply as a backdrop to human activity and agency, in these four studies a notion of environment was adopted which allowed exploration of person–environment interactions. This approach parallels the work of other scholars who have researched older people's interactions with their homes and neighbourhoods and theorized the role of person–place interaction across the lifecourse and in society generally (for example, Rowles 1978, 2000; Lawton 1980; Bourdieu 1984; Laws 1984; Rubenstein 1989; Lefebvre 1991).

Movement and mobility

a day trip is alright, but more than that, you have got to think about toilets and all sorts of things. (Respondent, Study Four)

Fundamental to the discussion that follows is the idea that environment is never experienced as unitary or monolithic, but as a series of settings where people experience their day-to-day lives. It can be conceived, perceived and lived (Lefebvre 1994) as segmented, insofar as people's capacity for moving around allows them to enact different sets of behaviours in different categories of place. It is, at the very least, composed of an anchor point – perhaps a favourite room, or even a chair – from which the person can venture forth to other places (Kellaher 2002). This might simply be a different room or another chair; or places reached easily or with difficulty. Some people become temporarily or permanently unable to make such moves without assistance. Here the interaction between personal mobility and social environment becomes crucial. Such trips may, though, become no longer possible at all, so that there is only the anchor point and no destination point to permit a travel trajectory to be conceived. The evidence suggests that, notwithstanding strategies to engage with other worlds through people, thoughts, books and other media, identity and QoL are likely to be impoverished relative to life before such limitations in the individuals ability to move around (Study One).

Aspects of the material environment that could act as barriers had become significant to older people in each of the four studies. Traffic flow, street gradients and kerbs, levels of dilapidation and vandalism had some influence on getting out and about. On top of this, health and access to transport affected how these barriers were experienced and dealt with. For some people in these studies, personal movement had been affected by sensory losses. For others, ageing had heightened the sensual impact of the micro-environment so that ground textures, changes in level, and physical barriers had become problematic. With age, people needed places to pause, and sit, and to visit the lavatory. Poor morale became increasingly prevalent with worsening mobility. In Study Three, regardless of social class, people in the worst quintile of mobility had eleven times the odds of those in the highest quintile for poor morale. The following observation from a woman, aged 77 (Study One), illustrates how reduced mobility impacts upon social activities and the sense of self:

I live my own life, I can't say I don't get lonely, I do. I miss [my husband] to this day, and I don't think I will ever get over that. And . . . so I have to keep myself as occupied as I can, so what do I do? I am very fortunate to have a mobility scooter, which I couldn't afford, but I said to myself at the time 'What is more important, the money in the bank or your QoL?' and I came up with the answer that obviously life is more important, so I went for it and I bought it. And I have never regretted it, and it means I can get out and enjoy myself.

So, I go out and . . . I come [to a club] on a Monday and I go out on a Thursday and call the bingo [laughs], yes. And I am in the play reading group and I visit a lot of elderly friends in their homes. And, I always seem to be doing something, going into town, doing shopping, or I had a friend here who has unfortunately gone, and we used to go and do things, go out on trips, but not as much as I used to because I am getting more lame unfortunately. I think I need to go out mostly. I don't mind having a day in from time to time and being quiet. In fact, sometimes I welcome it. But . . . occasionally, you know, you get days when you feel down and . . . I try to cope, I am inclined to be a depressive at times and especially in the winter when the weather is bad, and I have to have pills to keep me up [laughs]. I don't mind my own company, I have usually got something to do, and if I have got nothing to do, I have got a book, I can read, but you get fed up with reading. And I do think I am a social being, I am happier with small groups of people, rather than crowds, I don't like crowds at all.

I like to go on little outings, you know, and things like that. But I am restricted now, and that is a very difficult thing to come to terms with, not to be able to do what you want to do. It is awfully difficult. You have just got to accept it, and it is so hard, I find it so hard to accept. For instance, I put my name down for a trip, like we were going to go to Peterborough or something, so I put my name down straight off. And so I went home and thought 'I can't do that! I can't walk all that way, what are you doing?' and very often I do this, I put my name down because I want to do everything and then I have to realize that I can't. It is like when you go on a bus trip and you come through a nice little village, and you think 'this will be a nice place to come and visit one day with a friend' and then you realize, how can you visit the little place? You can't walk it.

Place, movement and morale

This woman's experience demonstrates that getting out and about is very much a QoL issue. Not surprisingly then, having to stay in bed was associated with poor morale for a significant minority of people aged over 75 in Study Three. As shown in Table 4.1, six out of nine components of the mobility score contributed to the morale score. These components related to a range of mobility options, reflected in the other studies, and were moulded by personal, social, and environmental attributes. The most extreme mobility limitation, 'staying in bed most of the time', was omitted from the calculation of morale because less than 1 per cent of this sample had such a serious limitation. For four of the components, however, substantial numbers of people said that the limitation on their mobility was not due to their health and the two groups ('health' and 'other reasons') were analysed separately. For 'staying at home most of the time', 'staying away from home for short periods', and 'not getting about in the dark', poor morale was more likely if the mobility limitation was due to health, rather than if it was not.

Study Three found that overall prevalence of poor morale was lowest in rural areas, with differences between rural and non-rural areas in the relationship

Table 4.1 Associations between components of the mobility score and poor quality of life

Component of mobility	Prevalence (%)		Odds ratio for poor morale[1]	p-value
	Men	**Women**		
Only get about in one building	5.2	11.0	1.06 (0.8, 1.4)	0.59
Stay in one room	0.9	1.3	2.10 (1.3, 3.3)	0.003
Stay in bed more	15.5	14.4	1.84 (1.5, 2.2)	< 0.001
Do not use public transport now				
– because of health	13.4	28.1	1.08 (0.9, 1.3)	
– for other reasons	24.6	16.3	1.04 (0.9, 1.2)	0.61
Stay at home most of the time				
– because of health	23.9	36.3	2.66 (2.2, 3.2)	
– for other reasons	31.7	24.7	1.49 (1.2, 1.8)	< 0.001
Only go out if there is a lavatory nearby	16.8	18.2	1.79 (1.5, 2.1)	< 0.001
Do not go into town	14.9	20.0	1.12 (1.0, 1.3)	0.12
Only stay away from home for short periods				
– because of health	20.1	28.3	1.34 (1.1, 1.7)	
– for other reasons	25.6	22.0	1.16 (0.8, 1.6)	0.05
Do not get about in the dark or in places that are not lit unless I have someone to help				
– because of health	16.5	27.9	1.75 (1.4, 2.3)	
– for other reasons	25.2	43.8	1.41 (1.1, 1.7)	< 0.001

Note: 1. Adjusted for gender, age, marital status, living alone, social class, population density and the other components of mobility listed. Also takes into account clustering within general practice.
Source: Study Three.

between mobility and morale. In both rural and urban locations staying at home for reasons to do with health increased nearly threefold the odds of having poor morale. In rural areas, staying at home for reasons other than health (compared to not staying at home) did not significantly affect the odds of having poor morale. In non-rural areas, however, the group who stayed at home for reasons other than health had a 60 per cent higher chance (95 per cent CI 26–108 per cent) of having poor morale than those people who did not report a limitation. In rural areas it made a substantial difference to the odds of poor morale whether or not 'only staying away from home for short periods' was due to health reasons or not (respective odds ratios –1.5 (1.0, 2.3) and 0.7 (0.4, 1.1)). But in other areas, where both health and other reasons for limitation were associated with increased odds of experiencing poor morale (respective odds ratios 1.3 (1.0, 1.6) and 1.3 (0.9, 1.9)).

These data are cross-sectional so we cannot establish whether poor mobility or morale came first. As social class predicted both mobility and morale, one possibility is that lower social class was a risk factor for poor mobility and this in turn accounted for class differentials in the chances of poor morale. In particular, being limited to staying in one room most of the time, or to staying in bed, carried double the odds of having poor morale. Staying at home was also an adverse factor, but more so if attributed to health problems – perhaps less controllable than opting to stay at home.

In Study Three, 'not using public transport' was not a factor in poor morale, nor was 'not going into town'. However, the environment and facilities outside the home could be important, as evidenced by the increased risk of poor morale if excursions are deterred by poor availability of lavatories or unlit places. However in Study Four, not using public transport was often associated with using private transport, which in turn was associated with better QoL. There are other possible explanations for the findings in Study Three, for example, incontinence might account for both poor morale and needing to know there is a lavatory; or poor sight might account for reluctance to go out in the dark and poor morale. This still leaves the rural areas advantaged with respect to morale. There may be some self-selection in that those continuing to live in these areas can cope and find ways of enjoying life without travelling far; and differences between rural and non-rural social environments need also to be considered and further researched.

Morale, neighbourhood and change

Study One found that both the broad structure and the fine detail of environments affected how people could use the area local to home. The material complexity of the neighbourhood, whether it was rural, suburban or inner-city, mattered to people. Familiar places, especially those where people had long-standing connections, could support older people in a number of ways including underwriting an entitlement to place by virtue of co-history of habitation; conferring the security of knowing and being known by other people, even if only by sight; and the confidence of knowing how to manage the material environment – good places to cross the road, public lavatories, short-cuts, safe routes, and special places. To some extent familiarity could also compensate for losses in hearing, sight, and so on. Respondents could also feel supported or undermined by the status of their immediate neighbourhood relative to neighbouring areas.

Whatever the size of a person's effective neighbourhood, a comfort zone of interest and control can be proposed that fades away from the intimacy of the home base, the loss of control made steeper by disability or frailty. In neighbourhoods experiencing troubles, the gradient may become steep for almost everybody. The speed of decline experienced in some areas presents a crucial challenge to the ability of older people to assimilate neighbourhood change. In recent years, socially deprived areas are likely to have experienced physical deterioration of the housing stock or local landmarks, and the loss of the various public and commercial services. Such areas are also characterized by relatively high rates of population turnover, and those who live in them are disproportionately vulnerable to a range of crimes (Social Exclusion Unit 1998):

> It has changed, you get difficult people coming to live here and it gets very dirty, when I first came over here the roads were clean, now the roads up there are untidy. (Woman, aged 69, Study One)

> That's why we don't know anyone, because they're coming and going. They change. They're just hopping from one house to another and we don't really know a lot of people in the street now. As I say, we've lived here 38 years. But they're in transit, aren't they? They just live there, then go. (Man aged 63, Study Two)

> [It] is not safe if you leave your house. It might get broken in. In the early days, you used to be able to go to the sea – six months, seven months – and you would leave your house empty and it will remain safe. I mean if you leave for half an hour now, you might come back and see they burgled the house. (Somali man, Study Two)

When taken together, the features of deprived urban neighbourhoods can interact to reduce the well-being of older residents. Coming to terms with neighbourhood change presents a particular challenge to older people who have lived in a particular area for a long time and witnessed decline which has affected their patterns of movement. For example, in relation to the loss of services, older people may need to leave their own neighbourhood to reach shops, a chemist or a post office. Concern about crime – discussed further below – might mean that some people will not leave the house alone or will have to rely on taxis to get around. High population turnover may disrupt individuals' abilities to maintain stable social relationships, confounding many older people's desire to be surrounded by those similar to themselves (Cattell and Evans 1999). Not only do people feel protected when surrounded by those with similar attributes (Phillipson et al. 1999), but they may feel more secure when living among those with histories broadly parallel to their own. Such natural groupings may differ from collective living within settings such as 'sheltered housing', which though experienced as more secure, may exacerbate segregation and obstruct integration with neighbourhoods if boundaries between home and neighbourhood become rigid.

Socializing

Basically my neighbourhood is these flats. I mean, I know everybody. (Man aged 61, Study One)

I went out shopping this morning along the bungalows, and a lady was coming along and she said 'Good morning'. And I've never seen her before in my life. People are friendly. The majority of them are. (Woman aged 81, Study Two)

In Study One, important parts of people's day-to-day social activity took place in their own neighbourhood, especially if they did not have a car. Being part of a community in this way appeared to give people confidence that they could get help if they needed it. Some people had reasoned that at a particular stage in life they had to decide to settle and make wherever they were at that time their home and community for life. Such strategies give rise to different levels of involvement with the neighbourhood, related to personal disposition, circumstances and health.

In Study Two, many older people identified local family, friends and neighbours as features of their neighbourhood that they liked. This finding was supported by data on involvements in a range of informal social relationships that suggested a high level of movement in and around the immediate locality. Of those respondents with children still living (81 per cent of the sample), a quarter (26 per cent) reported sharing a house with a child, a further 22 per cent had a child living within one mile of their home, and 24 per cent had a child living between one and five miles away. Many respondents without children, or who had children living further away, had other relatives living close by. For example, 41 per cent of those with siblings (76 per cent of the sample) had a brother or sister living within five miles of their home. Such proximity to members of their family has a significant influence on the frequency of older people's family contacts. More than one-third of respondents (34 per cent) saw a relative every day, and a further third (32 per cent) saw a relative at least weekly. For two-thirds of older people in these deprived areas, therefore, there was a regular and fairly intense level of family contact. A minority maintained less frequent contacts with 9 per cent indicating that they saw a member of their family on a fortnightly or monthly basis and 11 per cent reporting less frequent contact. Fifteen per cent of respondents reported having no children or relatives, or never seeing them.

Contact does not of course mean the same thing as personal mobility, although each has a bearing on the other. Being visited at home, for example, may mean that an older person with very poor mobility can get help to move from room to room or from chair to chair, or to get out of the house. Social participation and engagement have been identified as a critical element in the QoL of older people (Victor et al. 2003), and although research shows older people experiencing loneliness or isolation to be in the minority, the persistence of habitual and later-life loneliness continues to have implications for policy and practice. Social interactions both inside and outside the home, as initiated by the older person and by others, contribute to the dynamics of interactivity implied in 'getting out and about'.

Many older people in the deprived areas of Study Two were in regular contact with friends and neighbours. Almost four-fifths of respondents (79 per cent) could identify at least one friend in their local community. Of those with friends, almost half (47 per cent) had a chat or did something with a friend every day. A further 29 per cent got together with friends two or three times a week, and 17 per cent saw friends at least once a week. Only 8 per cent saw a friend less often than this. Contacts with neighbours were slightly less frequent than with friends, but also fairly common. Two-fifths of older people saw a neighbour to chat or do something with every day, and a further two-fifths saw a neighbour at least once a week. Some 17 per cent of respondents lacked contact with neighbours altogether or saw their neighbours less often than once a month.

Transport

> In the normal way I would walk down for the benefit of my health, and then take the bus back from the bus station. (Man aged 84, Study One)

I find that Stratford is good because I can walk to Stratford, do my shopping, walk home and don't have to worry about buses. I can get to Ilford from here. I can get to Romford from here. And if you're aged you get a bus pass in Newham. You don't get it everywhere . . . The station is quite near; you can get to most anywhere from Stratford Station. I like living here. (Woman aged 65, Study Two)

Many older people continue to use combinations of transport, including walking, in the areas immediately around their homes; but for those continuing to move in and out of the neighbourhood, car ownership and access to public transport are significant issues. Some people, especially current older generations of women in Britain, have never had independent access to a car, and as men and women age, they are increasingly likely to give up driving. Compared to younger adults, and especially if they live alone, older people are less likely to own cars. This reflects not only more limited financial resources in many cases, but also a range of other practical difficulties such as finding a parking space or securing a vehicle against damage or theft, which may make car ownership just too bothersome. In Study Two, just 26 per cent of older people had access to a car. This means that for many older people, moving out beyond the neighbourhood requires accessible public transportation, taxis, or the help of others. Reliance on others for transport in particular may diminish for some the sense of control over movement/mobility that can be crucial to self-esteem and the perception of what is possible and practical.

Study Four found that access to transport generally, and car ownership, were associated with higher perceived QoL, independent of wealth. Convenience, flexibility, and comfort were the most mentioned benefits of car ownership, and for some people having access to a car was seen as a life-line because it enabled them to get out of the house. Car ownership was seen as allowing a 'fuller life', or as a means of extending the range of viable accessibility (Studies One and Four); indeed, some respondents in the latter study suggested that 'you build your life round the car'. Car ownership appeared to be more important to QoL for men than for women. In Study Four, car ownership and driving were seen as associated with independence, although concerns were often expressed about rising maintenance costs – especially as people got older – and about potentially failing health and the safety of continuing to drive. It seemed that a decision to give up driving could be made harder by other aspects of driving mentioned by many, such as enhanced self-esteem, status, social role and identity, retaining a valued skill, and the ability to offer lifts and be of service to other. Hardly surprisingly, the prospect of giving up the car is anticipated with a deep sense of loss. However, those who had given up their car were more positive in their views about living without it, compared with those who were still driving (except in relation to saving money). The study found that taxis were perceived as expensive and tended to be used only on 'special occasions'.

For people with minimal access to a car, even as a passenger, arranging lifts could be an issue. Whereas most people might be able to get a lift 'as and when needed', it was clear that arranging it could often be awkward. Many respondents in Study Four expressed great reluctance to ask for a lift, preferring to be 'independent', even of their own adult children, who would 'have their own lives'. Independence in this context could variously mean not going after all, taking a taxi, or where feasible, taking public transport.

Travelling by public transport is a social activity, regarded positively by some respondents – 'you can have a blether on the bus' – but negatively by many worried about the behaviour of other passengers, or disliking mobile phones, smoking and litter. In Study Four a number of respondents expressed concern about personal security when using public transport, especially at night. Table 4.2 gives an indication of the barriers perceived as most important when using public transport.

Barriers to the use of public transport can stem from people's increasing frailty as they get older, combined with characteristics of the transport itself.

Table 4.2 Ten most frequent barriers for respondents aged over 70 years, with the proportion of that age-group who reported each as a 'problem'

Problems	% aged over 70 who agree
Personal security in evening and at night	80
Public transport running late	68
Having to wait	68
Difficulties carrying heavy loads	66
The possibility of cancellations	66
Behaviour of some passengers	64
Lack of cleanliness	54
Having to be out in bad weather	54
Having to change transport	53
Difficulties travelling where I want to	50
Difficulties travelling when I want to	48

Source: Study Four.

Problematic aspects of public transport, such as unreliability, difficulties with access and costs, were often compounded by decline in the level of service in some areas. Despite concessionary fares, there are a number of ways in which public transport is not 'age friendly'. Although all these factors can have an impact on the lives of older people, the finding that the most cited problem was concern about personal security after dark reflects a more diffuse barrier to older people being able to get out and about as they would wish.

In Study Four, anticipated problems with getting about, including having to give up driving, were associated with negative perceptions of old age, so that most people said they could not bring themselves to actively plan for such eventualities. Yet many older respondents in the study expressed ambiguity about continuing to drive in the face of rising costs and potentially failing health, especially when public transport could provide an alternative that was often less stressful, and which was acknowledged by many as environmentally preferable. It is then, a matter of concern that some bus and train operators regarded older passengers as a 'nuisance' rather than as customers. Many of the barriers to the use of public transport, for example, lack of cleanliness, inaudible announcements and lack of information, could easily be tackled. The requirements of older passengers must be taken seriously within an integrated travel policy, and we argue that doing so would improve services for the whole population.

Security

> We don't go out at night. Unless we are in the car, we wouldn't dream of it. And you wouldn't walk through the town at night. (Man aged 63, Study One)

> Well, I used to take the dog for walks of a night. But there's that many kids around here. They're terrible, the youths. They're not nice. (Woman aged 63, Study Two)

Respondents in both urban and rural locations in Study One reported insecurities about going out at night, but people living in the city, more than in rural areas, had concerns about their personal safety during the day. Their main worries were about crime, especially drug-related crime; lewd or other unacceptable activities in public places; excess traffic, noise and litter; and street disturbances. While some ascribed these problems, in part, to the increasingly multi-cultural composition of their neighbourhoods, most felt that the main problem was with younger people, including children and young families as well as teenagers and young adults.

Older people in deprived areas are much more likely to experience crime than those in Britain as a whole (Scharf et al 2002). Not surprisingly, this translates into fears about becoming a victim of crime and restrictions in movement around the neighbourhood. The overwhelming majority of older people taking part in Study Two indicated that they would feel unsafe going out alone in their neighbourhood after dark, with only 7 per cent feeling very safe. Concern about personal safety when out alone after dark was more evident among people aged 75 and over than among those aged 60 to 74 years. Over half (56 per cent) of women reported that they would feel very unsafe alone in their neighbourhood after dark compared with 28 per cent of men. Other studies have found similar differences: in the 2001 British Crime Survey the respective proportions were 33 per cent of women and 9 per cent of men aged 60 and over (Kershaw et al. 2001: 75).

Most older people who are concerned about their safety when out alone in the evening will tend to avoid leaving their home after dark. In this respect, it is important to emphasize that a majority of older people in deprived areas tend to feel much more secure when they are in their own homes at night. Overall, 46 per cent of respondents in Study Two felt very safe and 41 per cent felt fairly safe in their own homes at night. Just 4 per cent indicated that they felt very unsafe. Responses to this question did not vary significantly according to a person's gender or age, but one in ten of Indian, Pakistani and Somali older people reported feeling very unsafe in their homes at night, and were rather less likely to feel secure in their own homes after dark than those describing themselves as white or Black Caribbean.

Conclusion: the importance of getting out and about

By creating neighbourhoods that are suitable for people of all ages and reducing crime and the fear of crime, all residents in an area, not just older people, could feel more secure and would be more likely to engage with their local communities. This continues to be an issue in area regeneration. In Study Two, the analysis of patterns of social interaction with local family, friends and neighbours, and the impact of crime on daily life showed the ambivalent relationship of older people to their (deprived) urban environment. On the one hand, there was evidence of a high level of movement to and from the houses of other people residing in the locality. On the other, such movements could be restricted by the justified concerns of older people about their personal safety beyond the home. This inevitably has an effect on social networks, and policy should recognize the importance of informal social relationships in sustaining local communities.

Bringing together data from studies within the Growing Older programme has allowed ongoing 'indefinite triangulation' of data from studies across the spectrum of qualitative and quantitative methodologies (Fielding and Fielding 1986). By combining data from our four studies, the importance of environmental aspects that are material, social and psychological can be shown to impact upon 'getting out and about'. In this way the importance of characteristics such as social class, gender and ethnicity can be seen as accentuating issues including security, social interaction, mobility and accessibility. All these factors contribute to the possibilities and limitations of engagement in later life.

People need to have access to domestic and neighbourhood environments that permit the real possibility of ringing the changes. We have seen how morale slumps for the minority of older people confined to one space – the bed or bedroom – and we know from earlier work that the single-cell represented by the residential room is rarely sufficient for a person to reveal – to self and others – the complex individual that has emerged from many decades of experience (Willcocks et al. 1987). Older people appear to accept, albeit reluctantly, considerable limits on the distances they may cover and their identity is not necessarily threatened as long as there remains some room for physical and cognitive manoeuvre. The implications for policy are that the QoL and well-being of older people can be crucially enriched and extended by attention to the environment and the opening up of opportunities for people to get out and about.

5

Family and economic roles

Lynda Clarke, Maria Evandrou and Peter Warr

Introduction

Individuals undertake a variety of social and economic roles over the lifecourse, including those of spouse, parent, grandparent, carer and paid worker. This chapter examines the experience of taking up such roles and discusses the social and economic exchanges which take place in different environments. Research findings are included from three different ESRC Growing Older (GO) studies. Both quantitative and qualitative methods are employed, and data are analysed from a cross-sectional and lifecourse perspective using some of the concepts introduced in Chapter 2.

First, we discuss the theoretical frameworks found useful in the analysis of the empirical data. Then findings from a project on grandparenthood are reported, outlining the types of grandparental roles, the associated activities and constraints, and the impact upon quality of life (QoL) in old age (Clarke and Roberts 2003). Combining family and economic roles brings benefits and costs to individuals and families at all stages of life. The next section summarizes the GO study investigating psychological well-being in jobs and retirement (Robertson et al. 2003). The results of a third GO study, examining multiple role responsibilities, are then discussed (Evandrou and Glaser 2002a), and a concluding review examines some implications from these investigations.

Theoretical background

The evidence on multiple role commitments is largely based on North American studies, focusing on the relationship between multiple role responsibilities and health and well-being. The research reflects two opposing theoretical perspectives, the role strain hypothesis which proposes a negative association between multiple role obligations and well-being (Goode 1960), and the role enhancement hypothesis which suggests that occupying multiple roles may have a positive effect on well-being (Sieber 1974; Marks 1977). In general, empirical evidence suggests that those with multiple roles are more likely to be in better physical and mental health (Adelman 1994a, 1994b; Voyandoff and Donnelly 1999), and to engage in more social activities (Farkas and Himes 1997). On the other hand, some studies have demonstrated either higher levels of reported psychological strain among women with multiple roles (Beck et al. 1997; Jenkins 1997), or little or no effect of multiple role commitments on various measures of well-being (Verbrugge 1983; Spitze et al. 1994; Penning 1998; Reid and Hardy 1999).

This variation between findings is likely to reflect the fact that it is not only the number of roles that matters, but also their content. For example, undertaking a paid job in addition to being a family carer can introduce attractive new opportunities (for social contact or increased income, for instance), but also present challenges and potential threats (e.g. through an excessive load of personal demands). The value of multiple roles thus depends on their characteristics. A set of key environmental characteristics is considered later.

Causal interpretation of findings in this area is not straightforward, and a simple pattern of influence from role incumbency to well-being should not be assumed. For instance, it is often important to consider self-selection into a role. Positive associations between role membership and subjective well-being may reflect the fact that role incumbents with higher well-being have chosen to enter the role, whereas people with lower well-being have chosen to avoid it. It is therefore important for research to ask about personal preferences which may underlie role selection, and a GO study of that kind will be summarized later.

Older people's QoL is also a function of the role they play within the family. Family links and intergenerational solidarity may be crucial in contributing to many older people's well-being and for the avoidance of social exclusion. In Bowling's (1995) investigation of QoL, relationships with family and relatives were named as the most important aspect, well ahead of anything else. In a GO study of individuals aged between 50 and 74, family activities were particularly associated with both life satisfaction and affective well-being (Warr et al. 2004). These relationships encompass emotional, practical and financial support as well as feelings of reciprocal obligation.

Intergenerational exchanges work in both directions (Quereshi and Walker 1989; Aldous 1995). Older people can usually rely on care from their children, but where both parents are working or where family breakdown has occurred, grandparents may be expected to care for grandchildren or to contribute to their support in financial or emotional terms. The consequences of family breakdown and particularly the loss of contact with grandchildren can be severe for the physical and emotional health of grandparents (Kruk 1995). These issues are further explored in relation to an ESRC GO study in the next section.

Family roles and quality of life in old age

Family relationships are central to the well-being of individuals, family groups and society in general. These relationships encompass emotional, practical and financial support, as well as less tangible feelings of mutual support and reciprocal obligation. While relationships with partner, children and parents may be most important for younger adults, relationships with grandchildren are also relevant for older people. Yet, there is very little information in Britain about relationships between grandparents and their grandchildren.

In its Consultation Document *Supporting Families* (Home Office 1998), the Government endorsed the valuable role that grandparents play in supporting families and stated that it wanted to encourage grandparents to play a more positive role in the lives of their families. However, it may be as misleading to generalize about grandparents as about older people, as the research evidence from the USA suggests that there is a large degree of diversity and heterogeneity in grandparenting roles. One of the main aims in the ESRC GO study of grandparenthood (Clarke and Roberts 2003) was to examine the nature of grandparental roles and to establish the extent and nature of grandparents' financial, practical and emotional support for their children's families. The project also explored whether grandparenthood contributed to the QoL of older people and the extent to which current grandparenting roles, levels and types of activity are chosen by, or constrained for older people.

The study employed both qualitative and quantitative methods to investigate these issues. In the first stage, a telephone interview of a national sample of grandparents was conducted by the Office of National Statistics (ONS) in 1999/2000, which was repeated and extended in 2001. In Stage two, 45 grandparents from the national sample were interviewed in-depth on the meaning and activities of grandparent roles. In Stage three, information was collected on intergenerational help between grandparents and grandchildren. The main advantage of the ONS survey data over previous British data is that it documents grandparental roles in relation to all sets of grandchildren, rather than just some.

Grandparenthood and quality of life

Grandparents were unanimous in reporting that grandparenthood was an important part of their life. Most (70 per cent) rated the relationship with their grandchildren as 'one of the most important in my life' and a further 15 per cent said it was 'the most important'. Over half (55 per cent) of the respondents reported that being a grandparent contributed 'enormously' to their QoL, about a third (31 per cent) said it contributed 'a lot', and only 4 per cent stated it did not contribute at all.

The grandparents participating in the in-depth interviews were also asked about the importance of the grandparent–grandchild relationship, followed by an exploration of which other relationships were important to them. Seven out of 45 respondents stated that the grandparent–grandchild relationship was the most important in their life and nine that it was an important relationship but not central to their lives. As in the survey, the majority of grandparents stated that their relationship with grandchildren was one of the most important in their lives. For these grandparents, other important relationships were those with children, grandchildren and family generally, and for those who were married or with a partner, their relationship together was singled out. Friends were also mentioned by the respondent as being important.

The grandparents were also asked which three factors had increased the quality of their lives. Relationships with family members, including children and grandchildren were mentioned the most often (28 out of 45). Good health was the next most frequently mentioned factor (13), followed by their relationship with their spouse or partner (9). Having sufficient money was also mentioned (8). Other factors believed to increase their QoL (in order of importance) were: friends, being able to do things, work, holidays and being a member of a church/having faith. The factor most frequently mentioned as decreasing QoL was their own ill-health or that of others (17), followed by financial worries (6), work stress (4) and not being able to get around (4). Other factors mentioned included worry about family, being alone and living in a bad neighbourhood. As above, relationships with other family members were overwhelmingly identified as the most important factor in increasing QoL.

There was only one respondent in the study who reported that being a grandparent had detrimentally affected his QoL. This grandfather had taken on the care of his 2-year-old granddaughter following his daughter's increasing drug problem. Although he represents the only case where a decrease in QoL was reported, his position is worth reporting, particularly as very little is known about custodial grandparents in Britain compared to the USA (Fuller-Thompson et al. 1997; Casper and Bryson 1998). Taking on the care for his granddaughter had a major impact on the life of the respondent, and not a fully positive impact. He strongly felt, however, that he wanted a relationship with his granddaughter, whatever personal sacrifices he had to make. When asked how his life had changed he said:

> I don't want to use the word burden but, yeah, it's changed my life and not for the better . . . If I hadn't stepped in and done this, she would have been adopted and I wouldn't have seen her, and that's why I stepped in and took custody. It wasn't ideal but then again, I want to see my grand-daughter so in a way I wouldn't say I've ruined my life but I've basically put, it's like, putting your life on hold, you know, for what is going to be ten, fifteen years, I don't know.

Grandparents and family support

Without adequate, nationally representative data there has been a tendency in public policy to ignore the diversity of grandparents' circumstances, roles and obligations. The government has emphasized the importance of grandparents for family life through caring for children when mothers work, as well as providing support when families break up or experience difficulty. To this end it has urged local housing authorities to enable wider family members to live near each other whenever possible (Home Office 1998). In the GO study, information about grandparents' provision of help and support was obtained in the qualitative interviews. The findings highlighted the variation between grandparents in what they provided, how they helped and what they were willing to do for their families. There was considerable diversity in what people felt was appropriate. Most grandparents were generally prepared to step in to 'help' their children with the grandchildren when needed; for example, with childcare, babysitting or with help in times of family break-up or a crisis. While some were clearly prepared to 'drop everything for the grandchildren', others wanted time for themselves and set boundaries on what was legitimate or not. 'I've told them to count me out unless they are in real trouble . . . I'm not a built-in baby sitter . . . if there's a crisis then they know I would help.'

Three main types of support were identified: practical, financial and emotional. Grandparents, particularly grandmothers, historically have played and still play a key role as an additional source of childcare and are routinely used for practical support in times of normal upheaval, like the arrival of new babies, moving house and illness of parent, but they have also taken on a key role in more protracted crises. Some reported having a separated child and family return 'home' and found this difficult over a long period. Others stepped in to give practical help when the loss of a partner made practical life more difficult for their child and grandchildren. Some grandparents were providing extensive help and time looking after their grandchildren, particularly where the mother worked. At the extreme was the grandfather mentioned earlier, who had taken on the custody of his grandchild.

Generally, practical help was seen as part of the relationship, although some grandparents indicated that they had no choice about the amount of childcare they provided. They described their daughters or daughters-in-law as having to work to pay the rent or mortgage and there being no other way to find childcare that the family either could afford or find acceptable. Some grandparents resented this, but viewed their inconvenience as the lesser of the two evils.

The study found that financial help and support varied enormously by both the income level and values of the grandparent and circumstances of the child. Some grandparents went out of their way to buy many 'extras' and luxuries for their grandchildren: 'we've bought bikes for them . . . they've had music centres . . . we bought their Sky', others routinely helped with things more likely to be necessities 'I'm the one who gets the shoes'; other grandparents were upset that their own circumstances meant they could not do as much as they wanted; 'well, I can't buy her things and that hurts me'.

The experience of divorce and separation often meant grandparents stepped in to remedy financial difficulties. At times, it was viewed to 'even up' the experiences of cousins in intact families; 'we guarantee them a decent holiday, they can talk about it with their friends, . . . it keeps them up with their cousins' or more basic support for a lone mother or a daughter-in-law.

Emotional support in most families was found to be a constant dimension of the 'give and take' of family relationships. It was only commented on when it was recognized as above the level usually expected and this was particularly associated with family break-up. Many grandparents in this situation described how they both held back, tried not to take sides but saw a key part of their role as providing 'a stable platform for the kids'. Some grandparents were found to be even more involved in trying to help their very upset grandchildren: 'We was always being sent for in the night if anything was wrong . . . and if Joseph was a bit upset, which he used to be, he'd crying for his dad, we'd bring him home with us.' Overall, analysis of the grandparents' accounts indicated that they offered a range of support, most of it willingly, but sometimes less so due to a lack of an alternative source of help for their children and grandchildren.

Grandparenting: constraints and negotiation in the role

The role of grandparenthood is partly outside the control of the individuals concerned. The decision to have grandchildren is not necessarily something grandparents can influence. The middle generation controls whether the older person becomes a grandparent and, to a large extent, the nature of the interaction between the grandparent and grandchild. One grandmother summarized her feelings as 'being a grandparent is a privilege but it's not something you should grovel for'. Parents of children can act as 'gate-keeper' to their children and many grandparents were keenly aware of this. Indeed, negotiation of the grandparental role is a key theme in grandparents' discourse, as is the concept of 'not interfering'.

Nearly all the grandparents in the study's national survey were found to be involved with their grandchildren (only 0.5 per cent said they never saw their grandchildren) and were aware of needing to strike a balance between providing support and not saying or doing anything that might be perceived as interference by the parents in order to avoid conflict and tension. Most grandparents recognized the tenuous nature of their position and the necessity of 'standing back and letting the parents get on with the job of bringing up the children themselves'. Rather, it was the responsibility of grandparents to 'be there' to advise if needed or asked, be supportive and show an interest without being critical or 'overstepping the mark and interfering'. A number of respondents recognized that perhaps their behaviour had changed since their children became parents and that they should not comment on their children's parenting methods. Grandparents reported a number of strategies for ensuring an equilibrium between themselves and their children in order to maintain contact with their grandchildren.

Conflict between grandparents and their children about grandchildren, if it occurred, was reported more commonly when grandchildren were young. This was usually concerned with behaviour or parenting methods, particularly in relation to feeding. The feeling of a need to atone for arguments or disagreements on behalf of the grandparent revealed the insecurity of this role. Non-interference can be difficult to maintain especially when families part. Grandparents reported trying not to interfere in family conflicts but feeling obliged to step in to help their child if they felt close. This has been found in previous studies (Drew 2000) and is confirmed by the findings of the Cardiff Law School in their study of divorced families (Ferguson et al. 2004).

Some respondents said that the separation or divorce of their children did not have an impact on their role as grandparents. But many grandparents reported substantial changes to their own lives when children's families parted, not least in the amount and type of support they felt called upon to provide or the increase in tension they experienced in 'trying to be fair to/ keep in with all sides'. The separation or divorce of grandchildren's parents can make negotiation of the grandparent role even more fraught than usual and has severe repercussions, leading in extreme cases to a complete breakdown. While this is rare at present, it is feared and has a reality which shapes many grandparents' reactions. Given the recent increase in family separation, this will probably become more prevalent and, from the statistical analysis of the study's survey data, it is most likely that paternal grandparents will be the grandparents who have less contact with grandchildren after family break-up.

Economic roles: psychological well-being in jobs and retirement

Paid employment is central to western societies. Most adults spend much of their life at work, in a relationship that ends with a transition to retirement. Recent decades have seen a trend towards earlier retirement ages than previously, although some stabilization appears to have occurred lately. At present, some 70 per cent of British people are in paid employment between the ages of 50 and 64 (men) or 60 (women) (the state retirement ages). Above those ages, the rate is about 9 per cent.

Issues of work and retirement are important to older individuals personally, and also to government agencies because of implications for the funding of pensions and for national productivity. One concern is for possible differences in well-being, for example, because experienced well-being can influence people's motivation to seek or avoid a role.

Research has yielded varied results in that respect. Continuing in paid work has been found in different studies to be both beneficial and harmful compared to retirement, and often no difference has been observed. For instance, having a job after the formal age of retirement was accompanied by greater life satisfaction (compared to non-employed people) in research by Aquino et al. (1996), but findings by Reitzes et al. (1996) favoured older people's non-employment, and no difference was observed by Ross and Drentea (1998). This inconsistency is likely to arise in part from between-study differences in the age-ranges studied and in the definition of each employment-related category.

However, inconsistency between previous findings is likely also to derive from between-study variations in the environments experienced by study participants. For some individuals, retirement (or alternatively employment) carries with it desirable features, whereas for others in different circumstances those roles have mainly negative characteristics. For example, an older person with substantial caring responsibilities might experience distressing overload from the addition of paid employment.

A general model of the environmental characteristics that influence well-being (Warr 1987) covers situations of all kinds, and may be applied to the life-space of older adults. Based on studies of younger people's employment, unemployment and non-employment, the model proposes that any environment enhances or impairs happiness through the impact of nine key features (referred to as 'vitamins', by analogy with physical health). These are: (1) opportunity for personal control; (2) opportunity for skill use; (3) externally generated goals; (4) variety; (5) environmental clarity; (6) availability of money; (7) physical security; (8) opportunity for interpersonal contact; and (9) valued social position. There is considerable evidence that processes within each of those categories bear significantly on psychological well-being at younger ages.

One GO investigation into employment and retirement applied this model to individuals in the age range 50 to 74. It was proposed that each employment role (and also being unemployed and seeking a job, when below state pension age) would vary in its impact through the level of the key environmental characteristics. In that way, continued employment, for instance, could be either good or bad for an older person depending on the level of the characteristics; well-being in retirement might also depend on their level. The study thus assessed the nature of people's environments in each role, rather than merely comparing individuals in each category ('retired' versus 'employed'); QoL was expected to depend on environmental content, not merely on category membership.

Questionnaires were completed by 1167 British men and women aged between 50 and 74. Participants were identified as employed, unemployed or retired, and each person completed multi-item scales to tap perceptions of each of the nine environmental factors in their life as a whole. The outcome variables of interest were affective well-being and life satisfaction. Measures of life satisfaction are more based on reflective consideration of one's life to date (e.g. 'if I could live my life over, I would change almost nothing'), whereas affective well-being is more a short-term emotional state (e.g. feeling 'calm and peaceful', not feeling 'downhearted and blue'). Items in these scales are presented by Warr et al. (2004).

The environmental characteristics were found to differ significantly between the three respondent groups. Environments of older unemployed people were substantially impoverished in every measured respect, relative to those of both employed and retired individuals. In addition, workers in comparison to those who were retired reported significantly lower opportunity for control and significantly more externally generated goals, a higher quantity of interpersonal interaction, and a more valued social position.

Low environmental levels in unemployment were accompanied by significantly reduced well-being of both kinds; as in other studies, these older unemployed people had significantly lower levels of well-being than others. However, comparisons between employed and retired persons indicated that on average those two groups had equal life satisfaction and affective well-being. It seems appropriate to conclude (consistent with the variable pattern of previous findings illustrated earlier) that in general there is no great difference in happiness between being retired or being employed at older ages. Short-term transitional disruption might be envisaged, but, in general, happiness is likely to be similar across the roles.

However, patterns may vary between situations, and we need to consider possible moderating factors. For example, how closely were between-person differences in the nine key environmental features accompanied by differences in life satisfaction and affective well-being?

Correlations between perceived levels of the environmental characteristics and life satisfaction averaged +0.40 for individuals in the three roles; for affective well-being, the average value was +0.30. The level of these characteristics is thus significant in employment, retirement and unemployment at older ages, more so for life satisfaction than for affective well-being.

In order to examine in more detail the importance of the environmental features, hierarchical multiple regression analyses were carried out. As the first step, associations of life satisfaction and affective well-being with role incumbency were computed; as described above, unemployment was clearly harmful, but no differences were present between having a job and being retired. Next, the environmental characteristics were included in the analysis as well as each person's employment role. The pattern of combined association is set out in detail by Warr et al. (2004).

Consider the results for life satisfaction. Including in the second step of the regression analysis the nine environmental characteristics, as well as a person's role, removed the significant association with role itself. In other words, perceived features of the environment statistically accounted for the association between employment-related role and life satisfaction; it was the level of environmental features that mattered, not being in a particular role. The important features for life satisfaction in this study were opportunity for personal control, variety, environmental clarity, availability of money, physical security, quality of interpersonal contact, and valued social position. Life satisfaction was greater for older individuals experiencing more of those features than for others, whether they were employed, retired or unemployed.

These environmental characteristics were selected on the basis of previous research evidence that they are important for well-being. The fact that they were found to be associated with life satisfaction in this sample is therefore not surprising. The noteworthy finding is that differences in average well-being between employment-related roles are accounted for by the features. It is not being retired, or in any other role, that matters in the causation of well-being. The same characteristics of the environment are important in any role; in order to understand well-being in employment, unemployment or retirement, we have to ask about their level. Irrespective of a person's role, differences in these primary features account substantially for his or her well-being.

In addition to environmental features, a second possible moderator of well-being in employment-related roles is personal preference. Do people want to be in their current role, or is that forced upon them for financial or other reasons? Preferences in this area have sometimes been examined in terms of expressed commitment to paid work. During unemployment, a negative association has been found: people who more want a job when unemployed are even less happy than others (Warr et al. 1988). That was also found during retirement in the GO study described here. For retired individuals aged between 50 and 74, the correlations of employment commitment with affective well-being and life satisfaction were -0.25 and -0.30 respectively; retired people who more wanted to be in paid employment experienced less happiness. (For members of the sample who were in paid jobs, the correlations were positive; stronger employment commitment was associated with greater well-being.) Happiness in a role depends in part on one's wish to be in that role. The importance of personal preference is also shown in respect of a person's influence over the timing of his or her retirement. Swan et al. (1991) reported that individuals who had been required to retire, rather than choosing to do so, exhibited more depression and more negative feelings about being retired. In practice, many involuntary retirements occur because of ill-health, and greater health problems among involuntary retirees are likely also to contribute to their poorer subsequent well-being. In the GO study, early retirees who had been forced to retire because of ill-health reported significantly lower affective well-being and life satisfaction than did those who themselves chose to retire early.

The relationship between employment-related role and indicators of well-being thus depends on environmental characteristics and (linked to those) on individuals' preferences. We need to examine those more specific variables, not merely people's position in the labour market (retired, unemployed, etc.). Differences between published findings about retirement, illustrated at the beginning of this section, are likely to arise partly from unmeasured differences in these moderating variables. Furthermore, the variables can be expected to influence life satisfaction and affective well-being in a range of other roles.

Combining family and economic roles

Recent socio-economic and demographic changes, such as increasing female labour force participation, rises in the age at which children leave home and improvements in longevity are all likely to have increased the number of people 'caught in the middle' – that is, juggling paid work and caring responsibilities, while still supporting their own children. This section explores the extent of multiple role occupancy in mid-life (45–59/64 years) and investigates the relationship between multiple role responsibilities and QoL as measured by material resources. Data from the 1994–95 Family and Working Lives Survey (FWLS) were used to investigate current and past multiple role commitments and variations in the number of roles held. The FWLS is based on a nationally representative sample of 9139 individuals aged between 16 and 69 years in Britain, interviewed in 1994–95. A key advantage of the FWLS over the General Household Survey (GHS) is that it includes retrospective data on past episodes of caregiving, paid work and family life. Variables were derived for each month of the respondent's life from the age of 16 to their age at interview, indicating whether or not they had provided care, had children in the household, or were in paid work. This enabled us to determine both current and past role commitments.

The research focused on the occupancy of three roles: 'parent', 'carer' and 'paid worker' (Table 5.1). The partner role variable distinguished between those individuals who reported that they were living in a cohabiting or marital union and those who were not. The parental role variable distinguished individuals who had children of any age in the household (including adopted and step-children) versus those who did not, in keeping with previous studies (Spitze and Logan 1990; Rosenthal et al. 1996; Farkas and Himes 1997; Penning 1998). The literature confirms that the demands of dependent children are likely to be greater than those of adult children (Bartley et al. 1992;

Table 5.1 Operationalizing role occupancy and role intensity in the FWLS

Role occupancy	Role intensity
Carer	
Providing care to someone who is sick, disabled or elderly	Providing care for 20 or more hours a week
Parent	
Children of any age living at home	At least one dependent child or an adult child who is either: a) permanently sick, disabled or unable to work; b) unemployed; c) divorced/separated/widowed; d) at least one child aged 25 years and over living at home & no adult child contributing to household income
Paid worker	
In any paid work	Working full-time (over 30 hours per week)

Source: Evandrou et al. (2002).

Dautzenberg et al. 1998; Reid and Hardy 1999). Thus, those living with at least one dependent child were defined as having a more 'intensive' parental role.

Extent of multiple role occupancy

Analysis showed that being 'caught in the middle', in terms of simultaneous family and care-giving responsibilities while in paid work, remains an atypical experience. Only a small proportion of individuals in mid-life combined paid work with consistent caregiving or held other multiple role configurations. There were distinct gender differences, with men being equally or more likely than women to face multiple roles, reflecting their higher labour force participation and later timing of parenthood (Table 5.2). Demographic and social characteristics were found to affect the take-up of multiple roles, with greater age, being unmarried, and being in poor health all significantly reducing the likelihood of holding multiple roles among both men and women (Evandrou et al. 2002).

Although the proportion of individuals in mid-life who currently hold multiple roles of those examined is relatively small, when investigated over a longer time period the proportion is much higher (Table 5.3). In particular, a significant proportion of people have provided care at some stage in their lifetime. Thus, when examined over the lifecourse, multiple role occupancy

Table 5.2 Distribution of individuals in mid-life (45–59/64 years) by gender and various role combinations (%)

Current role occupancy	Men (45–64 yrs)	Women (45–59 yrs)
No roles	21.7	15.3
One role		
Carer	1.9	2.9
Parent	9.3	15.1
Paid worker	27.5	27.7
Two roles		
Carer, parent	0.8	2.2
Carer, paid worker	1.2	1.9
Paid worker, parent	36.2	32.4
Three roles		
Carer, parent, paid worker	1.4	2.6
N	(1330)	(1178)
$\chi^2 = 46.92$; DF = 7; $p = 0.000$		

Note: All sample numbers presented in tables are unweighted, whereas percentages given are weighted.
Source: Table 3, Evandrou et al. (2002).

Table 5.3 Distribution of mid-life individuals (45–59/64 yrs) by gender and retrospective multiple role occupancy (%)

	Men	Women	Total
Never had two or more roles simultaneously	13.1	7.9	10.6
Ever had two roles simultaneously			
Ever carer and parent	–	0.1	0.1
Ever carer and paid worker	2.8	3.7	3.2
Ever paid worker and parent	72.9	65.8	69.6
Ever paid worker and parent and (at another time) carer and parent	0.8	4.7	2.6
Ever had three roles simultaneously			
Ever carer and parent and paid worker	10.5	17.9	13.9
N	(1027)	(947)	(1974)
$\chi^2 = 63.92$; DF = 5; $p = 0.000$			

Source: Table 8, Evandrou et al. (2002).

is a much more common experience than cross-sectional analysis suggests, emphasizing the importance of taking a dynamic approach.

Impact of role occupancy on economic well-being

Previous studies have largely relied on cross-sectional data to examine the relationship between multiple roles and well-being (e.g. economic resources and health). In this project, extended life history information was used from the Family and Working Lives Survey to investigate the effects of multiple role commitments in prior years on pension entitlement in later life. The retrospective history information was used to derive measures of lifetime work experience. This facilitated the calculation of the average pension entitlement accumulated by each respondent and the investigation of how this varied according to current and retrospective role occupancy.

Welfare state benefits, in the form of National Insurance Credits (NICs) and Home Responsibility Protection (HRP) provide significant protection for those men and women who are providing care or who are a parent and not in paid employment. Once Credits are added to years of contributions through paid work and years of HRP are taken into account, there was little difference in overall entitlement to the basic state pension between different role configurations (Table 5.4).

However, there were significant differences with respect to entitlements to second-tier pensions (i.e. occupational and private pensions) (Table 5.5). As found elsewhere, women were found to be particularly disadvantaged (Ginn et al. 2001). Analysis of the FWLS found that 15 per cent of mid-life women had made no contributions to *either* a state or private second pension. The proportion increased to one in five (20 per cent) for those currently occupying one role as a parent. Just over half of mid-life women had contributed to an occupational or personal pension compared to three-quarters of men. However, among women occupying either a parent role alone or combining parenting with caring, this figure dropped to less than a third. Not only had fewer women contributed towards second-tier pensions, but they had, on average, also contributed for fewer years (13 years compared to 21 years for men). As the relative value of the basic state pension continues to decline, second-tier pensions will become increasingly important for maintaining an adequate income in old age. Given these findings, it appears that women who have fulfilled the important social roles of carers and parents look likely to continue to run the risk of being socially excluded in terms of financial resources in later life.

Table 5.4 Average entitlement to the basic state pension (as a percentage of full pension) accumulated over the lifetime to date among men and women in mid-life by current role occupancy status and age (FWLS)

	45–49	**50–54**	**55–59**	**60–64**
Men				
No role	64 (52)	77 (67)	82 (72)	91 (82)
One role: carer	72 (59)	77 (64)	85 (78)	96 (91)
One role: parent	73 (57)	72 (60)	88 (77)	97 (89)
One role: paid worker	69 (68)	78 (77)	88 (87)	91 (90)
Two roles: carer, parent	70 (65)	88 (82)	88 (69)	78 (61)
Two roles: carer, paid worker	71 (71)	69 (69)	81 (81)	97 (97)
Two roles: paid worker, parent	67 (66)	76 (75)	88 (87)	96 (95)
Three roles: carer, parent, paid worker	67 (66)	72 (72)	87 (87)	92 (86)
All mid-life men	68 (65)	77 (73)	86 (81)	84 (75)
[N]	[408]	[329]	[342]	[343]
Women				
No role	40 (28)	48 (40)	50 (43)	
One role: carer	56 (30)	54 (46)	55 (45)	
One role: parent	42 (28)	42 (28)	44 (31)	
One role: paid worker	48 (46)	41 (37)	42 (40)	
Two roles: carer, parent	45 (33)	61 (48)	53 (36)	
Two roles: carer, paid worker	49 (48)	60 (59)	43 (39)	
Two roles: paid worker, parent	39 (31)	43 (36)	37 (31)	
Three roles: carer, parent, paid worker	43 (31)	32 (18)	45 (41)	
All mid-life women	42 (33)	43 (36)	45 (39)	
[N]	[477]	[405]	[435]	

Notes: Based on main FWLS sample only. Mid-life defined as 45–64 for men and 45–59 for women. Sample sizes based on unweighted data. Average years of contributions calculated using weighted data. Level of entitlement to BSP for a man is calculated as: (Years of contributions + Years of credits) / (44 – Years of HRP), and for a woman as (Years of contributions + Years of credits) / (39 – Years of HRP). Figures in brackets calculated *before* Credits and HRP taken into account.
Source: Analysis of 1994/95 FWLS.

Parallel to the government focus on promoting the 'Work–Life Balance' (DfEE 2000), further analysis examined the effect of caring responsibilities upon work arrangements and their likely impact upon pension prospects (Evandrou and

Table 5.5 Proportion of people in mid-life with any of the different types of second-tier pension (over the lifetime to date) by current role occupancy status (FWLS)

	State second pension (Graduated pension or SERPS)	Private second pension (Occupational or personal)	Any second pension	(N)
Men				
No role	60	70	93	(388)
One role: carer	71	62	100	(32)
One role: parent	77	75	98	(97)
One role: paid worker	72	79	97	(456)
Two roles: carer, parent	68	69	100	(7)
Two roles: carer, paid worker	84	66	100	(18)
Two roles: paid worker, parent	73	83	98	(343)
Three roles: carer, parent, paid worker	79	100	100	(12)
All mid-life men	70	78	97	(1353)
Women				
No role	61	40	78	(243)
One role: carer	63	53	89	(44)
One role: parent	68	28	80	(142)
One role: paid worker	59	63	87	(415)
Two roles: carer, parent	74	30	81	(18)
Two roles: carer, paid worker	66	65	94	(30)
Two roles: paid worker, parent	71	60	90	(285)
Three roles: carer, parent, paid worker	77	42	84	(24)
All mid-life women	66	51	85	(1201)

Note: Based on main FWLS sample only. Mid-life defined as 45–64 for men and 45–59 for women. Sample sizes based on unweighted data. Proportions calculated using weighted data.
Source: Analysis of 1994/95 FWLS.

Glaser 2003). Combining paid employment with caregiving was *not* an option for a significant minority of women with caring responsibilities in mid-life in the FWLS. One in five mid-life women who have ever had caring responsibilities reported that upon starting caring they stopped work altogether, and a further one in five reported that they worked fewer hours, earned less money or could only work restricted hours. Furthermore, a lower proportion of men and women who stopped work as a result of caring were members of an occupational pension scheme than other groups; and among those who were, they had on average accumulated *fewer* years of contributions than their counterparts who continued working. This will have direct implications for their level of pension income in later life.

Conclusion

Findings from these GO studies have a number of implications for family and economic roles, as well as for well-being in later life. The evidence from the grandparenthood study has emphasized the complexity of family relationships, the diversity of experience and meaning of being a grandparent, and the important social, emotional and financial safety net they provide. However, what was also clear was that grandparenthood is characterized by negotiation and constraint. The government has acknowledged the colossal potential in the grandparental role, particularly with respect to caring or in time of crisis. However, government documents and policy thinking need to take on board the heterogeneity of circumstance among the grandparental roles and among the family circumstances of the grandchildren. What is clear is that further research needs to be carried out in this area in order to unravel the complexities of this important family relationship and how it varies with the recent, and ongoing, changes in family life. Family relationships are more complex today but grandparenthood remains an important family relationship for many older people in Britain.

The project on paid employment has suggested that there is no overall difference in life satisfaction or affective well-being between older people who have a job and those who have retired from the labour market. Those aspects of life quality arise not from role incumbency itself, but from two other sets of factors: (1) the nature of the environment that is experienced; and (2) a person's wish to be in that environment.

Environmental characteristics that are important to older people's well-being do of course include the availability of money. But influential other features that vary between particular settings include the opportunities available for a person to influence his or her life-space, the possibility of predicting future developments, and the nature of interactions with other people.

The second moderating factor, an individual's personal preference, is based partly on those environmental aspects (people prefer roles with a desirable content), but also derives in part from established attitudes and motives. For example, continued employment into older ages has different implications for individuals who wish to be in a job and for those who have been coerced into the role for financial or other reasons. National and local policies need to recognize these differentiating influences, where appropriate, avoiding simple assertions based merely on role titles.

Combining family and economic roles over the lifecourse is a much more common occurrence than if we consider the experience at one point in time. Furthermore, national research indicates that the likelihood of having multiple family and economic role commitments appears to be increasing across successive birth cohorts (Evandrou and Glaser 2002b). Many people providing care, particularly women, face both a 'wage penalty' – in terms of reduced hours of work or withdrawal from the labour market altogether; and a 'pensions penalty' – in terms of reduced entitlements to state pensions and private pensions.

There has been increased recognition of the importance of supporting individuals in juggling work and family commitments, reflected in the government's launch of the Work–Life Balance Campaign (DfEE 2000). However, many of the schemes funded have focused primarily on improving the balance between paid work and parenting, with little attention given to the demands of caring for an older dependant. Urgent attention needs to be given to extending employment schemes currently available in Britain. Schemes such as parental leave, time-off for dependants and long-term career breaks, which are offered to individuals with childcare responsibilities, should also be made available to those workers with adult or elder-care responsibilities. In addition to encouraging employers to adapt and develop workplace practices to support carers, the government could provide financial incentives for people with caring responsibilities to remain in the labour market.

For the foreseeable future, many women who have fulfilled the important social roles of carers and parents will remain dependent on the basic state pension (BSP) as their main source of income in retirement. The level at which this benefit is payable is therefore fundamental in ensuring an adequate income in later life. At present, individuals with no source of income other than BSP are automatically entitled to means-tested Minimum Income Guarantee (MIG). The Chancellor has promised that future values of MIG will be indexed to earnings. While the value of BSP remains linked to prices, the gap between MIG and BSP looks set to increase with the result that more individuals will fall into means-testing during retirement. Unless the New Labour Government begins to 'think the unthinkable', and increase the value of BSP and restore the link to earnings, many women will be consigned to an old age living on means-tested benefits.

6

Social involvement
Aspects of gender and ethnicity

Kate Davidson, Lorna Warren and Mary Maynard

Introduction

In this chapter, pathways into social involvement are identified, and the importance of understanding participation as an active and passive experience is elaborated. The key cross-cutting themes include health, resources and social networks and their impact upon the choices that underpin older people's lives as they age. One of the major driving factors behind our Growing Older (GO) Programme-funded projects, each exploring aspects of older people's participation, was the desire to unpack further such complexity of social involvement when aspects of gender and ethnicity, both separately and together are taken into account. A shared aim was to go beyond simple measurement of social capital to account for quality of activities and of social contacts and relationships (Coulthard et al. 2002) across gender and ethnic boundaries.

As this chapter demonstrates, social involvement takes place within a variety of contexts: spatially (from one culture to another), temporally (within any one culture over historical time) and longitudinally (through any individual's life course). Furthermore, differences in the quality and quantity of social participation may be related to gender, ethnicity and age, but also to class and regional variation. The chapter examines these differences by drawing upon findings from the three inter-related projects: *The Social Worlds and Healthy Lifestyles of Older Men* (Sarah Arber, Tom Daly, Kate Davidson, and Kim Perren); *Older Women's Lives and Voices: Participation and Policy in Sheffield* (Joe Cook, Tony Maltby and Lorna Warren) and *Empowerment and Disempowerment: Comparative Study of Afro-Caribbean, Asian and White British Women in their Third Age* (Haleh Afshar, Myfanwy Franks, Mary Maynard and Sharon Wray).

Background

There is a growing body of research exploring the relationship between participation and involvement and the quality of life (QoL) of older people (Walker and Hennessy 2004). Within the field of policy the emphasis has been on participative paths to decision-making and the crafting of more empowered 'customers' (Barnes and Warren 1999). For older people, so often defined by their relationship with welfare services, such an approach may fail to address the most important issues in their lives. Indeed, the relatively new addition to the health field of the concept of social capital represents recognition of the fact that health-related behaviours, for example, are shaped and constrained by a range of social and community contexts (Coulthard et al. 2002). Profiles of such contexts are often derived from survey-based data. For example, in 2000/1, a social capital module, commissioned by the Health Development Agency (HDA) and incorporated within the long-standing General Household Survey (GHS)[1] asked about relationships and networks impacting on health in local communities (Coulthard et al. 2002). Two more recently established surveys also placing social capital at the centre of investigation are the English Longitudinal Study of Ageing (ELSA); and the Home Office's flagship Citizenship Survey (CS).

Among the positive findings of these studies regarding 'active retirement' is confirmation of the continued strength of older people's social networks and social activities. The majority of older people have at least one or two relatives living nearby (Coulthard et al. 2002) and see relatives or friends at least once a week (Walker et al. 2003: Table 52), and just under four-fifths say they have a hobby or past-time (Hyde and Janevic 2003). More problematic are the continuing obstacles to, and the feasibility of, participation. For example, two-fifths of older men and women have no close relatives living near them (Coulthard et al. 2002). Compared with younger people, older people, especially older women, are more reliant on public transport (Walker et al. 2003: Table 51) and considerably more likely to report difficulties accessing local amenities (Janevic et al. 2003).

More immediate, however, is the issue, which remains whether findings are positive or negative, of the extent to which we can understand participation through measurement alone. ELSA has certainly begun to fulfil its declared aim of filling in some of the gaps in the variable picture of what it means to grow old in the new century (Marmot et al. 2003). Nevertheless, other findings from ELSA and various of the surveys still leave us with numerous questions. Focusing on gender differences, we may ask, for example:

- ◆ Why is it that older women are more likely than men to report having a 'satisfactory relatives network' (Coulthard et al. 2002),[2] despite no significant differences in terms of seeing relatives?

- ◆ Although the differences are not huge, why is it that older men are more likely than women to be members of social clubs and to read newspapers but less likely than women to be involved in an education, art or music group (Hyde and Janevic 2003) and, with increasing age, to listen to the radio (Matheson and Summerfield 1999)?

Of equal significance are survey findings relating to ethnicity. While far fewer in quantity and rarely broken down by age and gender, they nonetheless consistently suggest differences in experiences of people across different ethnic groups which bear potential implications for older men and women. What are the meanings of trends which show, for example, Asian and Black adults to be more likely than White adults to be in regular touch with extended family members (a cousin, aunt, uncle, niece, or nephew) (Summerfield and Babb 2004) but less likely than White adults to have a satisfactory friendship network (Coulthard et al. 2002) or to report trusting people in their neighbourhood?

An additional weakness with the analysis of these surveys is the tendency to generalize the responses of sections of the population which incorporate huge diversity, not least in terms of chronological age. Qualitative studies within social gerontology, sharing the theoretical focus on 'participatory', 'active' or 'productive ageing' (Walker and Maltby 1997), have emphasized the notion of social quality and the identification of conditions which enable older people, as citizens, to participate in the social and economic lives of their communities in ways which enhance their well-being and individual potential (Beck et al. 1997).

The three GO projects

The main aim of the older men project was to examine the extent to which age, gender, marital status and former occupation influence choices and constraints in active and passive, private and public social involvement. Here, Kate Davidson focuses on men's individual participation within the family and social organizations. Lorna Warren broadens the remit to examine the social involvement of older women from different ethnic groups within a policy, framework in a society which rarely harkens to the voice of older women and even less to those belonging to ethnic minority communities. Mary Maynard strikes a positive note from her collaborative research on ethnic minority White and Black women who have largely adapted to living in the UK and for whom faith is an important link between their homeland and their adopted domicile.

Researching older men's social participation

Older men were the focus of the project carried out by Sara Arber, Kate Davidson, Kim Perren and Tom Daly between October 1999 and August 2002 (Davidson and Arber 2004). It is well documented that men are less likely than women to have extensive social networks in later life (Davidson et al. 2003) but little is known about the social dynamics of older men's lives.

Older men and social interaction

There was a widely held belief by the 85 men interviewed in this project that women (wives, mothers, daughters, nieces) played a pivotal role in the establishment and maintenance of wide social networks. Older men enjoy and maintain close relationships, although the scope and intensity vary according to marital status. Within the four categories of older men interviewed: married, widowed, never married and divorced, issues of continuity and discontinuities are important in understanding current social involvement.

The married men reported large, stable social networks, primarily (but not exclusively) couple orientated. In widowhood, these networks contracted and the men tended to rely more heavily on their adult children for support. Divorced men who reported more attenuated relationships with their adult children, tended to seek another close companionship (which did not necessarily involve sexual intimacy). On the other hand older never married men, who had established few close relationships in younger years, did not seek intimacy, and did not report feeling deprived, but they did see themselves as 'different'. They described themselves as 'loners', 'individuals' or 'completely independent':

> I'm a proud individualist . . . I don't seek a lot of human company, I never say anything profound, I don't need someone sitting there particularly. I've never felt this great yearn for companionship. (Jeremy, 71, never married)

It could be argued that those who do not particularly seek companionship reflect the concept of 'desirability' or choice of limited social networks. It is difficult to judge whether these men are more solitary because they do not seek social involvement, or whether it is because other people do not, or never have, sought their company. The circumstances which mitigated against marriage, especially for men, included among others, physical disadvantage, personality traits and poor income prospects. However, a common prejudice is that 'loners' are less happy than gregarious people, but to see happiness as a function of people's orientation to their world is simplistic (Schaie and Willis 2002). The never married men, like Jeremy, who did not desire 'someone sitting there', were content with their own company. The divorced men, on the other hand, did not enjoy their reduced circumstances, including financial and companionship status.

Older men and community involvement

Unlike other forms of social attachment, such as involvement in family life or the world of work, informal group membership is nominally accessible to all. Most of the men interviewed were involved in some sort of social group outside the home. These ranged from social and sports clubs to religious groups and civic organizations (such as voluntary agencies, community groups and political parties). Some were overtly leisure-oriented while others appeared to be guided by a spirit of altruism, religious belief or shared principles.

Older men's involvement with formal associations represents an undervalued resource which may contribute to the QoL of older men by facilitating social interaction and providing a context for continued social productivity. While all facilitate social interaction, some additionally offer the opportunity to pursue a personal goal (such as health maintenance) or to make a recognized social contribution through community activity. The opportunity to be part of a socially productive organization may bolster the well-being of older men by compensating for some of the losses following retirement from paid work.

There were notable differences between the organizational activities of partnered, widowed, divorced and never married men. The never married older men were less likely to be members of an organization than those with a partner, apart from religious organizations. Compared with partnered older men, those who were widowed were more likely to be involved with sports and social clubs, perhaps indicating that leisure associations offer compensations following widowhood. This pattern was not evident for men who were divorced, who had the lowest level of involvement in 'any' organization and are particularly unlikely to be members of sports clubs or religious organizations. Interestingly, Utz et al. (2002) found that widowed men and women had higher levels of informal social participation than partnered persons, whereas formal social participation levels were comparable between the two groups. They suggest that social participation levels tend to decrease prior to the death of a spouse, primarily because of poor spousal health but increase after bereavement as a result of greater support from friends and relatives. However, the majority of their sample were female and as suggested here, there are gender differences in support systems both before and after bereavement.

The men in the highest social groups were more involved in sports clubs which are likely to promote physical health, and in civic and religious organizations which may include involvement in activities that are altruistic or benefit the community. This contrasted with men with a history of manual labour, who were more likely to undertake sociable leisure. This class disparity has implications for social policy initiatives directed at older people which seek to combine social interaction with some other 'benefit' such as enhanced physical health or community activities. There was no indication that lack of resources impedes membership of sports or social clubs, but there was a decline in membership with increasing age.

Friends and neighbours

The lifespan perspectives of Kahn and Antonucci's (1980) social convoy and Carstensen et al.'s (1997) socio-economic selectivity help capture the diversity and heterogeneity of older men's lives. After retirement from the paid workforce, men become more dependent on friends and neighbours for social interaction. As one set of friends, acquaintances and work colleagues move to the social network margins, others take on more importance. Positive neighbourly relationships offer sociability and the opportunity to give and receive practical support, which may be particularly important for older men who live alone. One key finding is that frequent contact with neighbours is not necessarily associated with greater neighbourly exchange of favours, particularly for older men living alone:

> No, not many close friends. I know my neighbours well. They're not friends but we get on extremely well together. But I've not really got any close friends round about here . . . My daughter is in touch two or three times a week, the other sons certainly telephone me once a week and I visit them both about once a month for lunch or something. (Kevin, 75, widowed)

The men who lived alone were less likely to give or receive favours than married men. For example, many of the married men helped widowed neighbours with garden chores, talking to workmen, giving car lifts for shopping, and so on. These favours were more often than not instigated by their wife. Widowed men reported a smaller circle of friends than when they were married, but they had maintained and in some cases strengthened, their relationship with their adult children and grandchildren. Divorced men in the sample were the least contented with their social situation and viewed the prospect of ill health and loneliness in old age with considerable anxiety:

> I'm not sufficient unto myself. I've never been a loner. I think one of the things I've always been terrified of all my life is not having a partner and finding myself like this. I'm sort of, kind of, gazing around saying 'How did it happen?' I know perfectly well how it happened. But no, that is something which rather terrifies me. I don't like thinking of it. (Jasper, 70, twice divorced)

Advanced age is one of the major determinants of reduction in formal social involvement. However, restricted economic resources and poor health also contribute to this decline. Interaction with family and friends is likely to be influenced by an older person's access to material resources, including car ownership, physical and mental health and degree of physical mobility. However, Arber, Price et al. (2003) found that the low level of social interaction with relatives and friends by divorced and never married men cannot be explained by any differences in age, lack of car ownership, disadvantaged housing tenure, or differences in physical disability. They conclude that marital history and continuity of close family involvement are more likely to influence the quality and degree of both private and public social involvement.

The older divorced and never married men had more restricted networks with kin, friends and neighbours. This lack of social embeddedness makes them more vulnerable to social isolation in later life. It is important for policy-makers to take greater account of the differentiation of older men according to partnership status. Policy is high on the agenda when considering social inclusion for a somewhat neglected group of ethnic minority women.

The following two sections are largely inter-related and discuss qualitative research carried out on White and ethnic minority older women in the north of England.

Older women's lives and voices (OWLV)

This study was undertaken by Joe Cook, Tony Maltby and Lorna Warren between January 2000 and April 2002 (Cook et al. 2004). A participatory project working with older women, a key aim was to raise awareness of issues affecting the QoL of older women across different ethnic groups and their involvement in services available to them.

Like the *Women, Ethnicity and Empowerment in Later Life* study, the OWLV project showed migratory history to be a major influence central to understanding many aspects of older people's social involvement and intimately linked with gender. Previous discussions (Cook et al. 2004) have noted the impact of their diverse experiences of migration on the QoL older women from different minority ethnic groups. Migration has affected health, resources and social networks in a number of ways which were often inter-related.

Family and social networks

Both the OWLV discussion groups and life-story interviews revealed the universal importance of family. Some women had taken on new roles providing childcare support for grandchildren concomitantly gaining a sense of self-esteem and usefulness. In contrast, a number of Somali and Chinese women who were not eligible to receive even a basic pension, spoke of a loss of independence and a sense of being a burden on their families. For some, the political or financial imperatives of migration had impacted severely on families.

Many Somali women were dealing not only with bereavement and issues of mental health as the result of the death of loved ones in the civil war (Cook et al. 2004) but also with finding themselves separated from close relatives and friends in the process of fleeing from the troubles and with the subsequent sense of displacement. One Somali woman, whose daughter was still in Somalia, commented:

> The worst experience was the civil war because I lost some members of my family and some are still missing. Due to the war I have experienced displacements. I have been separated from my daughter. (Somali woman, in her fifties)

However, while Somali women's social networks were irreversibly changed as a result of migration, the asylum they were granted in the UK was viewed positively – notably for some, in comparison with other countries – as opening up new doors to social networks. Some women spoke of new channels of involvement – if not for themselves directly, then for their children – and they identified extended family networks:

> When we came here in this country, we were welcomed and given the residence and we almost forgot the suffering we experienced at the camps . . . The children who are grown up here in this country and although they are not fluent in Somali language any more, they do speak good English. (Somali woman, in her fifties)

Downsides to the expansion of networks through children and their contacts related to issues of language. Differences of language and generational stake

(Jerrome 1996) meant that, even where received, informal support was not always effective or appropriate. Some Somali women spoke also of being increasingly unable to understand and relate to their own children (Cook et al. 2004) and noted the growing loss of the 'mother tongue' by younger generations. The reliance on children to act as interpreters in encounters with formal service providers was especially problematic. As one Chinese woman similarly observed: 'I have children who speak English, but they are not able to explain to me in Chinese in a way that I can understand.'

Employment and inclusion

Even when women had not migrated for reasons of asylum, for those women arriving in the UK without paid employment, achieving social involvement seemed more difficult as well as being hazardous:

> He [husband] sent for me from the [West Indies] . . . but then eventually when I was eight months pregnant he deserted me with the children, which was very difficult. (Black-Caribbean woman, 52)

At the same time, while a number of the Chinese older women had taken up work in the catering industry – typically in family take-away businesses – on arrival in Sheffield, employment in this instance did not guarantee involvement in social networks but, if anything, just the opposite. As other researchers have noted (Yu 2000), there is no identifiable China Town in the city and restaurants and 'take-aways' are dispersed thinly across the region. A Chinese woman spoke of long and demanding shifts which prevented most family members from socializing:

> There weren't as many Chinese people. I worked most of the time. I woke up in the morning, worked, then slept. (Chinese woman, 70)

An Irish woman spoke, in contrast, of training as a nurse in the UK and the way in which this both helped her to adapt to her new life and offered a degree of protection from discrimination:

> When I was old enough I went and trained to be a nurse, and, of course, as you realize . . . there was a very big [Irish] contingent of nurses in this country . . . and so because there were so many of us you didn't feel – and a great many of the Sisters and people like that, they were [Irish] so there was a different feeling all together about being [Irish] then. (Irish woman, 65)

For another Irish woman, however, her job made constraints to social involvement clear:

That was the awful thing, you felt ashamed because you had so much prejudice . . . you couldn't get on if you had a very pronounced Irish accent, you know . . . you weren't considered somehow good enough, you see? (Irish woman, 65)

The work-based prejudice experienced by the Irish respondent above, alongside other participants, mirrored and subsequently reinforced longer-established and wider prejudice. A number of the White older women who had been born in Britain voiced the kind of racist attitudes currently directed at minority ethnic groups. They claimed there were:

. . . too many people coming into this country now that's not paying anything. All these refugees and all these people, if they, if it's genuine but there's some trying to get in that's not genuine and yet they go and they get money but they've never paid a penny. (White British-born, 87)

Opposition to migrants and their effect on the economy is not new: a Black-Caribbean woman reported standing up to accusations of taking jobs from British-born people:

But I say to them I don't come on banana boat, my husband is over here. And my husband send for me and I come over on the plane . . . The Queen sent to Jamaica government to request people to come over here and they not going to make us stop coming to work or anything . . . understand? (Black-Caribbean woman, 77)

Health and social involvement

For some of the women migrating from hotter climates, the difficulty of adjusting to the British weather was of initial impact on their health, compounding difficulties in becoming involved:

The weather was different. It was very cold, I could not speak English. My health deteriorated and I found extreme difficulty to adapt to the new environment. (Somali woman, in her fifties)

. . . believe me sister, I was poorly, chilblain, fever, cold, I didn't come out of bedroom for months! (Black-Caribbean woman, 69)

Women across all groups acknowledged the broader embodied relationship between health and ageing (Bytheway and Johnson 1998) and described the efforts they made at making the connection a positive one at the level of personal identity (MacDonald and Rich 1984) and, subsequently, social involvement. Indeed, asked if her income prevented her from doing things, one 85-year-old woman replied: 'No, my body does.' The worsening of her rheumatism over a number of years had gradually prevented her from pursuing previous interests such as knitting and dancing, both of which played an important role in her relationships with others in her social network:

> Well, I can't knit now with my hands going, otherwise I would have kept all my children and grandchildren all in knitted. I used to do knitting, but my hands don't let me knit now so I'm reading anything. But my eyes are getting a bit weak . . . Oh, I used to love dancing. I did it until I was 70 odd. Well, when I was 80, I went with my daughter to line dance, but it was a bit too much . . . I am losing my confidence a bit now. (White British woman, 85)

Her loss of confidence had also made the participant in question 'terrified to death' of going out at night. Like many older people in general, she had responded to her declining social activity by 'downsizing' and focusing on other popular past-times: 'I just get comfy with the television.'

Findings from the OWLV project helped to illustrate and explain the importance of extended networks – family and other – in the lives of older women from minority ethnic groups, especially where those women were not in positions in paid employment (generally a resource in involvement). Women from all groups showed skills and abilities in adapting to changing patterns of and possibilities for social involvement. However, mechanisms still need to be put into place to support involvement at the social and also more political levels. For example, the findings reinforce calls for adequate help with translation and interpretation for minority ethnic older women (Cook et al. 2004), in areas of personal correspondence as well as in welfare-related issues.

Empowerment and disempowerment: a comparative study

The research team comprised Haleh Afshar, Myfanwy Franks, Mary Maynard and Sharon Wray. The research on which this contribution draws was based on interviews and focus group discussions with women from a range of ethnic groupings, including White British, African Caribbean, Asian and Polish women. A variety of religious affiliations was represented and included Protestant, Catholic, Hindu, Sikh and Muslim.

Despite coming from a range of ethnic backgrounds, there was, as in the OWLV project, general agreement among most of the participants that good health is the most important issue in relation to quality of later life, even more so than income. This has also been confirmed by other research (Farquhar 1995; Sidell 1995; Bernard 2000). Further, the majority agreed that retaining their health and agility was significant to their sense of autonomy, of maintaining control and agency in their lives and to their social involvement and participation. Key themes which emerged were those of being able to 'get around' and of 'keeping going'.

Being able to walk and to get out to the shops was extremely important for most of the participants, since this was regarded as a way of having day-to-day social contact and keeping in touch with neighbours and the local community. This social involvement was somewhat curtailed for many of the Indian and Pakistani women, due to language barriers, and they tended to have more geographically restricted social interaction as a result. The other women, however, reported a wide range of interests: gardening, swimming and dancing were regularly mentioned as activities with which women were involved. However, a clear distinction emerged between the majority of women, including those who were White and living in the inner city, and more affluent White women who had relocated to rural areas on their, or their partners', retirement. These latter women were much more active in voluntary and organizational work, for instance, the Women's Institute, heading walks for the local Ramblers' Association and providing a trolley service at a local residential home.

When interests were under threat due to ill health, many women spoke of their attempts to maintain their activities and keep active. Although they reported having a range of health problems, such as heart disease, high blood pressure, arthritis, diabetes and asthma, the women said that they felt positive about themselves and were not prevented from enjoying life. Overall, this group of ethnically diverse older women tended to continue their engagement in activities *in spite of* their health problems. Difficulties with mobility, for instance, were treated as challenges to be overcome, rather than inevitable hindrances.

Kith and kin relationships

The significance of relationships with family and friends for older women's perceptions of their social involvement has been raised in previous research (Phillipson 1997; Phillipson et al. 2001). Indeed, there has been criticism of the assumption that older people will, necessarily, be dependent on their families, that this is always a problem and that independence should be sought at all costs (Arber and Evandrou 1993; Friedman 1997). Instead, emphasis is increasingly being placed on the idea of interdependency and the role that obligation and reciprocity can play in older people's lives. In this research, participants can be broadly divided into two groups. On the one hand, were the minority ethnic and those White women, who had kin close by. The minority ethnic women, in particular, were often surrounded by extended family, as well as having family overseas. The White women, in both inner city and rural locations, tended to have lived in the vicinity all their lives. On the other hand, there were the more affluent White women, who through internal migration within Britain, were separated from family and previous friendship networks. This meant they were rebuilding new networks and bases of support, in which church, clubs and shared leisure interests were important.

Across all the ethnic groups, women spoke about having a 'purpose' in life as being a central element in them feeling that they were active social participants. 'Purpose' refers to having a clear set of roles or functions to perform and, for those whose family lived nearby, it was frequently the main source of their feelings of social involvement. As one African Caribbean respondent commented:

> . . . it makes me feel in authority because even now they're still coming to me for advice, you know? I'm not a person who interferes in their business I just leave them to do their own thing. But I'm always there. An' I make sure I'm there for them. I've got fourteen grandchildren an' I'm 73.

Similarly, a Polish participant said about her family that 'we all work together'. It is possible to think about the relations that many of our older women, whatever their ethnicity, have with their family in terms of a 'moral economy of kin'. This refers to the agreed tasks, obligations and reciprocal actions which bind members together. For instance, many of the minority ethnic and the less affluent White women offered a service to their children by looking after grandchildren, often stepping in when parents were at work. This was seen as both rewarding and as making a contribution to socio-economic relations, which would be repaid with money, with goods in kind or in the future when the women might become more needy. Asked about her childcare activities, one Dominican respondent replied that she was involved,

> . . . three days a week. Sometimes two, sometimes one. I've got five and I've had them all. So this is the last one so I might as well finish the job.

Another Dominican participant who had recently been widowed suggested that looking after her granddaughter was helping her cope with her bereavement. She said:

> Well, you know, I do like looking after her because she's a little gem . . . Because if I have to get up at six o'clock or seven I have an incentive . . . otherwise I feel sorry for myself and stop in bed. I enjoy it. I don't have time to remember anything.

Some of the African Caribbean women spent so much time caring for their grandchildren that they had almost become professional grandmothers. This was so significant to the economy of the extended family that they had to take the children with them when they attended their local elders' community centre. For this reason, they were suggesting that a crèche should be provided there. However, it should also be said that not all of the women relished an extensive commitment to grandparenting. Some of the African Caribbean women made it clear that they needed time off from such duties in order to visit friends and do other things.

It was also clear that, for many minority ethnic women, the existence of local community centres provided an important avenue through which they could meet friends, share language and culture and sometimes see satellite television from their country of origin. A Polish contributor referred to her local centre, for example, as constituting her 'life'. Centres based on ethnicity are important in terms of sharing identity, ethnic food, history, experiences and communal celebrations. This is a particularly important source of social involvement for women who may feel isolated by their inability to speak English.

The importance of faith and spirituality

A final important strand in older women's social involvement and participation is through religion. Religion is largely ignored as a resource for older people. However, it was highly significant for the women in this research. Many of the affluent White women attended church and were actively involved in its associated activities. Of the remainder, most attested to some kind of inner faith or spirituality. For most of the minority ethnic women, though, religion was integral to their lives. For many, faith and identity are deeply associated and language is an intrinsic part of worship and of relating to God. As one of the Polish women put it, 'You can speak to God in your own language.'

Barriers to public worship

Because religion is so important in these women' s lives, it is important to consider the likely effect of failing health or disability on their ability to use it as a form of social participation. Ainley et al. (1992) found that health has a mediating role in active religious participation. Although the majority of our participants enjoyed degrees of able-bodiedness, it was evident that, with increasing age and decreased mobility, a growing minority were finding themselves excluded from what had been a mainstay of their lives. Ill health or disability may also prevent some women from fulfilling their daily personal rituals. For example, one Muslim participant explained how, since religion is her main interest, she used to spend her time reading religious books but that her eyesight is now too bad to allow her to do so.

However, although these dimensions of faith are all important to minority ethnic women, there is a second aspect which also must not be dismissed. This involves a spiritual dimension, the possibility of having an inner life and sense of being and involvement in relation to God, which need not be connected with the material world. Sapp (1987), for example, has criticized the literature which exists on spirituality and ageing for placing too much emphasis on what people do. It is important to recognize that people's sense of connectedness and notion of self in relation to faith should not only be measured in terms of their active behaviour. For the minority ethnic women in this research, faith was a significant part of their day to day lives, offering hope, meaning and a sense of peace and well-being.

Conclusion

In this chapter we looked at choices and constraints, pathways and barriers to social interaction on the micro and macro levels: that is, both with kith and kin and in the larger community. They are not mutually exclusive as there are individuals who do not have access to close family networks as a result of geographical location, marital and fertility status, for example, and there are older people who, through ill health or lack of resources, have close family, but have restricted access to community participation.

Qualitative examination of the pathways and barriers to social participation helps to take us beyond the mere measurement of social capital to a much fuller understanding of factors enhancing but also limiting the extent and quality of social involvement when age, gender and ethnicity are at the centre of investigation. The three projects discussed here demonstrate the value of qualitative enquiry through asking questions of older people who are rarely heard: older men and ethnic minority older women.

Kate Davidson found that class and marital status were pivotal in influencing men's kith and kin and community socializing. Divorced and never married men have the smallest social networks and are the least likely to participate in community activities. Lorna Warren identified the centrality of community and belonging and efforts to overcome barriers of language within a familiar cultural context. Faith, whether extrinsic, as expressed in public worship, or intrinsic, as experienced in private, individual spiritual resources played a very important part in the lives of the women interviewed for Mary Maynard's project. Increased longevity means older people, and older women in particular, are more likely to experience grandparenthood for a longer period and have greater opportunity for involvement in the lives of their growing grandchildren than in previous generations. Thompson and Walker (1987) have described one role of grandparents as the 'lineage bridge': the span connecting the other two generations. In both these projects on ethnic older women, it is revealed that the lineage bridge also works to span cultures. However, there also can be a clash of cultures between grandparents and grandchildren and this is more evident in Asian and Chinese families.

All three projects revealed that health in later life is an important factor in community participation but that ill health does not necessarily preclude social interaction. Rather, it changes the nature and extent of participation. As our findings indicate, there are relatively few older people, regardless of gender or ethnicity, who lack any source of social capital and are subsequently completely socially isolated.

John Donne (1572–1631), metaphysical poet and churchman, famously wrote in his Meditation XVII, 'Devotions upon Emergent Occasions' (1623):

> No man is an island, entire of itself every man is a piece of the continent, a part of the main if a clod be washed away by the sea, Europe is the less, as well as if a promontory were, as well as if a manor of thy friends or of thine own were any man's death diminishes me, because I am involved in mankind and therefore never send to know for whom the bell tolls, it tolls for thee. (Donne 1990: 344)

The Meditation highlights the stark awareness of mortality as a fact of life but also proposes that people do not live in isolation and that all 'mankind' is interconnected. Contemporary understanding of 'mankind' encompasses gender and multi-ethnicity and differential lifecourse experience in a global dimension and thus Donne's meditation continues to resonate in the twenty-first century context.

Notes

1 The General Household Survey was run for the first time in 1971. It consists of two elements: the continuous survey and trailers or modules which are included each year to a plan agreed by the sponsors of the GHS.

2 Those who were described as having a 'satisfactory relative network' were those people who saw or spoke to relatives at least once a week and had at least one close relative who lived nearby.

7

Social isolation and loneliness

Christina Victor and Thomas Scharf

Introduction

A key dimension of current thinking concerning the promotion of quality of life in old age relates to notions of social engagement and social inclusion. Research has consistently demonstrated a strong and positive relationship between social participation, especially within kin and wider social networks, and a high quality of life. Older people consistently report that the social environment, especially social relationships with members of their family, is integral to notions of quality of life (Bowling 1995 and Chapter 2). This gives rise to the observations of Rowe and Kahn (1997) who suggest that a high level of social engagement is a key factor in achieving the goal of 'successful aging'. Furthermore, they argue that, with advanced age, the social context, in combination with the physical environment, exerts a more potent influence upon the experience of ageing than intrinsic genetic or biological factors. Hence manipulation of the social environment by, for example, interventions to promote social engagement and combat loneliness may offer pathways for the improvement and enhancement of quality of life in old age.

This link between social engagement and quality of life is not new. The 'activity theorists' of ageing similarly argued that the key to a good old age was the maintenance of high levels of 'activity', including social participation and the maintenance of kin and friendship-based relationships. While the prescriptive strictures of activity theory may have been replaced, the social environment exerts an important influence upon and context within which people experience old age (Bowling et al. 1991).

Given the centrality of the social environment to quality of life, there is a concern to promote social engagement among older people that is evident in policy-makers' interest in such themes as social capital and social exclusion. In a striking parallel with the term 'community care', notions of social capital and social exclusion manifest many different conceptualizations (Scharf et al. 2000; Smith et al. 2002). For example, the current social exclusion agenda has largely been defined in relation to the needs of the labour market, focusing upon those of employment age or those who will enter the labour market in the future (children and young people) (Scharf et al. 2004). Such a narrow conceptualization of exclusion is clearly problematic when it is examined from the perspective of older people: a group within the population that has largely been systematically excluded from the labour market. To address the circumstances of a broader range of population groups it is necessary to view social exclusion as a multi-dimensional concept that extends far beyond the narrow confines of the labour market, and potentially affects people of all ages. While there are a variety of different approaches to measuring exclusion, all include within their structure a dimension that relates to the 'social world' (Berghman 1997; Burchardt et al. 1999; Gordon et al. 2000). Hence Scharf and Smith (2004) have proposed that exclusion from social relations and civic activities represent two of the five key domains in their model of social exclusion in later life.

There are at least four different perspectives that could be adopted when investigating social participation and exclusion in later life (Townsend 1968; Andersson 1998). Peer group studies focus upon how social engagement and exclusion vary within a given age-cohort; age-related studies address ways in which social engagement differs within the same cohort as they grow older; generation contrast studies examine how social engagement varies between different age groups at the same point in time; and contrasting cohort studies compare the social participation of older people at different historical time points. There has been a concentration in research upon peer group studies in terms of empirical investigations of loneliness (de Jong Gierveld 1987; Holmen et al. 1992, 1994; Wenger et al. 1996), social isolation and exclusion (Scharf and Smith 2004). By contrast, other perspectives on exclusion and engagement have received relatively little attention.

It is evident from the literature that a variety of different terms and concepts are being used interchangeably to describe notions of social engagement, exclusion and participation. Social engagement is a diverse concept with different subdivisions relating to notions such as social capital, social participation and social networks. The predominant conceptualization of exclusion in terms of social relationships has been on studying the 'pathological' end of the distribution with a specific concentration upon isolation and loneliness. This largely reflects an approach to the investigation of social relationships in later life influenced by the study of 'social problems' and, perhaps, too ready an acceptance of the 'stereotype' that the normal experience of old age is of social neglect and reliance upon 'fragile' social networks.

In this chapter we are concerned with patterns of social relations and the civic participation aspects of (dis)engagement among older people living in the community. Although these dimensions are dealt with separately, we acknowledge the inter-relationships between them and their links with other dimensions of the social exclusion model developed by Scharf and Smith (2004): material resources, access to basic services and neighbourhood exclusion. However, while we are inevitably concerned with older people who may be viewed as 'excluded', we seek to locate these data within the wider context and examine the 'included' as well as the excluded.

Data sources

The empirical material for this analysis is provided by two studies supported by the ESRC Growing Older (GO) Programme. The first dataset is derived from a national survey of households in Britain (England, Wales and Scotland) conducted using the United Kingdom Office for National Statistics (ONS) Omnibus Survey. This is based on face-to-face interviews with approximately 2000 adults aged 16 years and over in their own home and undertaken monthly or bi-monthly depending upon demand. Researchers can purchase specific modules/questions on the survey or use it as a mechanism to identify eligible research participants, as was the case in this study. Respondents aged 65 and over participating in the Omnibus Survey were invited to participate in a 'Quality of Life' module that was administered at a second interview (see Victor et al. 2001; Bowling et al. 2002; Ayis et al. 2003). To control for seasonality and to generate a sample of sufficient statistical power, all the 1598 participants aged 65 years and over interviewed for the April, September, November 2000 and January 2001 Omnibus Surveys were invited to participate in the Quality of Life survey and 1323 agreed to do so. At follow-up 24 of these addresses were subsequently found to be ineligible, leaving a potential study population of 1299. Of this number 243 (19 per cent) declined to participate and 57 (4 per cent) were not contactable. This yielded a total study population of 999 respondents: a response rate of 77 per cent of those identified as eligible for the study and 63 per cent of those who participated in the index waves of the Omnibus Survey.

The second dataset is concerned with older people living in socially deprived urban neighbourhoods in Liverpool, the London Borough of Newham and Manchester. These areas represented the three most deprived local authorities in England, according to the most current official measure of area deprivation at the time of the research (DETR 1998). A programme of research was subsequently undertaken in the three most deprived electoral wards of each city, all of which were ranked among England's 50 most deprived wards in 1998. Recruitment to a survey phase of the research occurred in two ways. A first group of participants was randomly selected from local electoral registers using a coding classification based on individuals' first names. In all, 2302 individuals were selected, of whom 1116 were deemed ineligible to participate for one of the following reasons: they had moved house or died, they were the wrong age, or they were too ill to participate. Of the 1186 potentially eligible respondents, 360 refused to participate and 325 could not be contacted. Interviews were subsequently completed with 501 people aged 60 and over, giving a response rate of 42 per cent. One limitation of using a sampling method based on respondents' first names is that the approach is unable to identify people of the appropriate age who belong to some minority ethnic groups. To overcome this difficulty, and to generate sufficiently large samples from particular groups to facilitate statistical analysis, an additional sample of people belonging to the largest minority ethnic groups in each electoral ward was recruited to the study. This group was accessed through a range of community organizations and previously established contacts within the study localities. Some 99 older people of Black Caribbean, Indian, Pakistani and Somali origin were recruited by this method.[1] In order to achieve a higher degree of comparability with the Omnibus Survey, only those people aged 65 and over are included in the subsequent analysis (n = 456).

Sample description

The Omnibus Survey sample broadly approximates to the general population of older people living in the community in Britain. In demographic terms, this sample has significantly more men than the older population as a whole (Table 7.1). Rates of chronic illness approximate to national norms for older people living in the community, as do levels of social contact and material resources.

Table 7.1 Sample characteristics

	General Household Survey 2000/2001		Omnibus Survey 2001		Deprived Areas Survey 2000/2001	
	65–74 years	75 and over	65–74 years	75 and over	65–74 years	75 and over
Sex						
Male	47	38	52	51	43	37
Female	53	62	48	49	57	63
Marital status						
Single	6	7	6	5	9	8
Married / cohabiting	66	41	69	47	46	27
Widowed	21	49	18	43	33	60
Separated / divorced	7	4	6	4	12	6
% reporting long-standing illness	57	64	61	63	66	68
% reporting limiting long-standing illness	37	47	34	41	47	60

Sources: Walker et al. 2002; Victor et al. 2001; Scharf et al. 2002.

While not aiming to be representative of the general population of older people, the sample in the deprived areas study diverges from the national sample and that of the Omnibus Survey in several key ways. The proportion of female respondents aged 65–74 years is higher (57 per cent compared with 53 per cent), and the survey population includes a significantly higher proportion of widows than is found in Britain as a whole (33 per cent compared with 21 per cent at age 65–74, and 60 compared with 49 per cent at age 75 and over). Compared with national samples, respondents in the deprived areas survey were significantly less likely to be married or living as part of a couple. This particular sample is also more ethnically diverse than the general population of older people, reflecting the demographic profile of socially disadvantaged urban neighbourhoods and the project's recruitment strategy. Some 74 per cent of respondents described themselves as white, 13 per cent as Black Caribbean, 6 per cent as Somali, 3 per cent as Pakistani, and 4 per cent as Indian. The deprived areas sample is more vulnerable to poverty (Scharf et al. 2002), and shows higher rates of chronic illness than the general population of older people.

Social relationships in later life

Our aim is to establish patterns of social engagement among older people in contemporary Britain and thereby examine both levels of inclusion and exclusion in terms of the broad pattern of social relationships characteristic of older people within contemporary Britain. In considering this we need to address two key aspects that have informed much of the study of social relationships in later life: loneliness and isolation. However, before examining the 'problematic' end of the social engagement distribution, we locate these within the broader context of the general patterns of social and civic engagement that apply to older people.

Social engagement

Both surveys included broadly comparable measures relating to older people's involvement in a variety of informal social relationships. As Table 7.2 shows, levels of contact are high between older people and their families, friends and neighbours. Indeed, there is remarkably little difference in the frequency of such contacts between the two studies reported here and an equivalent national sample drawn from the General Household Survey (GHS). In all studies, contacts were most frequent with neighbours and least frequent with family. Around two-thirds of respondents saw members of their family at least once a week, and just over seven out of ten saw friends weekly. In the Omnibus and GHS samples, almost nine out of ten respondents reported at least weekly contact with neighbours. This rate was somewhat lower in the deprived areas survey (79 per cent). Our studies suggest, therefore, that older people maintain high levels of contact with a range of individuals. Moreover, these data are likely to under-report actual levels of social contact, since they do not include

Table 7.2 Levels of social contact with family, friends and neighbours (%)

	General Household Survey 2000/2001	Omnibus Survey 2001	Deprived Areas Survey 2000/2001
See family weekly	66	62	66
Phone family weekly	85	81	–
See friends weekly	70	71	72
Phone friends weekly	67	64	–
See neighbours weekly	88	89	79

telephone or electronic means of communication. In the Omnibus Survey, 81 per cent of respondents reported phoning a family member at least once a week, and 64 per cent were in weekly phone contact with friends.

It is, perhaps, instructive to compare these crude levels of social engagement with those reported in an earlier study. In his classic analysis of the social relationships of older people, Tunstall (1966) reported that 56 per cent of older people had seen friends in the week before interview and 53 per cent were in weekly contact with neighbours. These levels of social engagement are rather lower than those reported in our more recent surveys. While it is, of course, difficult to comment on how our samples valued these forms of social contact or how such 'meanings' may have varied over time, these data certainly do not support the proposition that older people have become less socially engaged over the past fifty years.

Civic engagement

Alongside participation in informal social relationships, the degree to which sub-groups within the population engage with religious or community groups or are involved in the democratic process represents an important strand within debates about social exclusion (Burchardt et al. 1999; Gordon et al. 2000). However, such debates are usually focused upon the disengagement from civic society of younger and mid-life adults. While our datasets do not always allow direct comparisons to be made in terms of forms of civic engagement, a range of indicators point to a relatively high degree of involvement of older people in more formal aspects of community life.

In the Omnibus Survey, over four-fifths of respondents (82 per cent) had undertaken at least one type of activity in the week preceding interview, and more than nine out of ten (93 per cent) had left the home during the same period. In relation to civic duties, 73 per cent of those taking part in the study had voted in the previous general election. Broadly similar findings arise from the deprived areas survey. Some 42 per cent of those questioned attended religious meetings at least once a year, and 33 per cent attended meetings of community groups. Using a list of 11 civic activities, 76 per cent of respondents had undertaken at least one type of civic activity in the past three years. The most commonly observed activity was voting, with 68 per cent having voted in the previous general election and 66 per cent in the last local election. Around one-quarter of respondents (24 per cent) had not participated in any of the listed activities. Taking attendance at meetings together with participation in civic activities, just 15 per cent of older people in deprived areas were not involved in some type of formal community activity. The fact that levels of voting and participation in religious or community activities were broadly comparable between the Omnibus and deprived areas surveys reinforces the findings reported above in relation to older people's participation in informal social relationships. Not only are most older people in Britain involved in relationships with family, friends and neighbours, but they also participate actively in central aspects of civil society.

Social isolation

Relatively frequent contacts with members of the family, friends and neighbours represent the norm for older people in the UK. However, some are prone to social isolation. This risk is likely to be greater for older people who have no children or other relatives, and can be reflected in the maintenance of irregular or relatively infrequent contacts with family members, friends or neighbours. In order to illustrate the degree to which respondents in both studies were prone to some form of isolation, we have generated a social isolation index that combines three characteristics (Scharf and Smith 2004). Older people who lack relatives or see family members less than once a week, who have no friends or see friends less than weekly, and who have less than weekly contact with neighbours are judged vulnerable to social isolation. Combining these characteristics produces a measure of isolation that ranges from zero (not isolated on any characteristic) to three (isolated on all three characteristics).

Applying this measure to the two sample populations produces strikingly different results (Table 7.3). In the Omnibus Survey, 19 per cent of respondents

Table 7.3 Levels of social isolation (%)

	Omnibus Survey 2001*	Deprived Areas Survey 2000/2001
None (score 0)	19	43
Low (score of 1)	45	37
Medium (score of 2)	31	15
High (score of 3)	5	5

Notes: Index based upon three characteristics: (1) has no relatives/sees relatives less than weekly; (2) has no friends/chats with friends less than weekly; (3) has chat/sees neighbours less than weekly. Range of score 0–3 (see Scharf and Smith 2004).
* Source: McCormick (2003).

were not isolated on any of the index characteristics and 45 per cent experienced low levels of isolation. Some 36 per cent of older people in this study were prone to medium or high levels of isolation. By contrast, older people in deprived areas were significantly less likely to be isolated. Some 44 per cent of those interviewed were not isolated on any of the individual index items and 36 per cent experienced isolation on just one indicator. The remaining 20 per cent were subject to medium or high levels of isolation. Interestingly, these data match individuals' own perceptions of isolation. When asked if they ever felt isolated from society, 20 per cent of respondents in deprived areas suggested that they did, with health problems or some form of disability being cited as the most common reason for feeling isolated.

These data suggest that the degree to which older people experience social isolation varies significantly according to the characteristics of their place of residence. While similar proportions in both study populations were prone to the most acute form of social isolation (isolated on all three characteristics), this affected relatively few people. However, the proportion of older people experiencing fairly intense forms of isolation (scoring two or more on the index) in the Omnibus Survey was almost double that found in deprived areas.

In the deprived areas dataset social isolation does not appear to vary significantly according to a range of individual characteristics. In particular, gender and age had little influence over the degree to which respondents experienced isolation (Table 7.4). Though not statistically significant, the levels of social isolation were highest among respondents who had never married, and lowest among those who were either divorced or separated. In the Omnibus Survey the link between marital status and isolation reaches statistical significance with the never married demonstrating the highest rate of isolation. This could reflect a 'real' difference or perhaps in some way be indicative of the smaller family networks of this group. The Omnibus Survey also demonstrates a link between isolation and the age and gender of respondents. Those aged 75 and over and men displayed higher levels of isolation than people aged 65–74 or females. While there are some parallels between the two studies in relation to the link between marital status and isolation, the differences outweigh any similarities suggesting that social isolation may vary according to characteristics of the local environment – a finding that clearly merits further research.

Loneliness

Loneliness is concerned with how individuals evaluate their overall level of social interaction and describes a state in which there is a deficit between the desired

Table 7.4 Social isolation according to participant characteristics (%)

	Omnibus Survey 2001			Deprived areas survey 2000/2001		
	No isolation	Low isolation	Medium / high isolation	No isolation	Low isolation	Medium / high isolation
Sex						
Male	18	42	39	45	36	19
Female	20	47	32	42	37	21
Age-groups						
65–74	23	46	31	48	34	19
75 and over	13	46	41	38	40	22
Marital status						
Single / never married	4	49	47	21	45	34
Married / cohabiting	21	44	36	44	36	19
Widowed	21	45	34	47	34	20
Divorced / separated	14	50	36	51	34	15
All	19	45	36	43	37	20

Sources: As Table 7.3.

and actual quality and quantity of social engagement. Following the approach adopted by de Jong Gierveld (1998), loneliness can be perceived as a multidimensional phenomenon comprising three different strands. The first and most salient element is a 'deprivation' component that relates to 'the feelings associated with the absence of an intimate attachment, feelings of emptiness or abandonment' (de Jong Gierveld 1998: 74). The second element concerns the time perspective, raising the question of the extent to which the state of being lonely might be prone to change. The third dimension incorporates a range of emotional aspects of loneliness, such as sadness, guilt, frustration and desperation (de Jong Gierveld 1998: 74). As such, this concept is distinct from being alone (time spent alone), living alone (simply a description of the household arrangements) and social isolation (which refers to the level of integration of individuals, and groups, into the wider social environment). While there is some commonality between these concepts, the overlap is unclear and the terms are not interchangeable (de Jong Gierveld 1998; Victor et al. 2000; Holmen and Furukawa 2002).

The two surveys used different methods to determine the extent of loneliness among older people. The Omnibus Survey employed a direct question, derived from the work of Sheldon (1948), that asks respondents to rate their level of loneliness (Victor et al. 2001, 2002). By contrast, the deprived areas survey used the 'indirect' 11-item de Jong Gierveld scale (de Jong Gierveld and Kamphuis 1985; Scharf et al. 2002). While the pattern of responses across the two studies is similar, the absolute levels of loneliness are rather different (Table 7.5). The highest proportions of respondents in both studies experienced no or little loneliness. In both populations, severe loneliness was experienced by only a minority of respondents with most older people not experiencing this severity of loneliness.

Table 7.5 Levels of loneliness (%)

	Omnibus Survey 2001		Deprived Areas Survey 2000/2001
Do you feel lonely?		De Jong Gierveld Loneliness Scale (range 0–11)	
Never	61	Not lonely (score of 0–2)	40
Sometimes	31	Moderately lonely (score of 3–8)	45
Often	5	Severely lonely (score of 9–10)	10
Always	2	Very severely lonely (score of 11)	5

Several factors might explain the observed differences between our samples in terms of the reported levels of loneliness. These explanations may be categorized as reflecting differences in methodology or sample composition. In relation to the former, the observed difference may reflect the under-reporting of loneliness when this is investigated by a direct and unambiguous question. Given the potentially stigmatizing nature of self-defining oneself as lonely, older people may choose not to define themselves in this way. They may not wish to compromise their 'public face' and either not report feeling lonely or 'down-shift' their loneliness rating. Alternatively, the very different nature of the two populations may offer a (partial) explanation. There is some support for the latter explanation in that a survey undertaken in Perth, Western Australia, using the de Jong Gierveld scale reported that 52 per cent were not lonely and 9 per cent were either severely or very severely lonely (Iredell et al. 2003). Furthermore, the highest rate of loneliness in a British study was reported at 16 per cent in a study of Hackney (Bowling et al. 1991). Taken together, these two pieces of evidence suggest that levels of loneliness, however measured, may be higher for older people living in deprived neighbourhoods and suggest that the neighbourhood environment can exert a strong influence on social engagement.

Who is most at risk of experiencing loneliness? The differing methodologies of the two studies permit only a limited exploration of this aspect. In the deprived areas study, loneliness did not appear to be related to age or gender (Table 7.6). However, there was a clear relationship with individuals' marital status. In this respect, respondents who were married were significantly less likely to be lonely than all other respondents. Loneliness was most acute among those who were single and had never married. Over one-quarter of older people in this category were prone to the most acute form of loneliness. In the Omnibus Survey loneliness was significantly statistically associated with increasing age and women were more likely to experience loneliness than men. As in the deprived areas study, the Omnibus Survey also showed a link between loneliness and marital status with the widowed at considerably higher risk of reporting loneliness than other groups.

Discussion

Comparison of findings from two rather different datasets shows that most older people in Britain are actively engaged in a variety of informal and formal social relationships. This is a general pattern that occurs in a variety of geographic locations. By contrast, relatively few older people are affected by

Table 7.6 Loneliness according to participant characteristics (%)

	Omnibus Survey 2001			Deprived Areas Survey 2000/2001		
	Never lonely	Sometimes lonely	Often / always lonely	Not lonely	Moderately lonely	(Very) severely lonely
Sex						
Male	71	23	6	40	42	18
Female	51	41	7	40	46	14
Age-groups						
65–74	55	38	6	44	43	14
75 and over	51	33	16	36	47	17
Marital status						
Single / never married	46	45	9	42	32	26
Married / cohabiting	78	21	1	50	43	7
Widowed	28	53	20	33	49	19
Divorced / separated	46	45	8	35	43	23
All	61	32	9	40	45	15

the most acute forms of social isolation and loneliness. However, the fact that a small proportion of older people experience intense isolation and are often or severely lonely warrants further attention.

Overall, levels of social isolation diverged considerably between the two samples. Older people in deprived areas appear to be less vulnerable to isolation than those in the population as a whole. However, the levels of severe isolation were approximately similar at 5 per cent and this is very similar to the levels reported by Wenger (1984) and Tunstall (1966). The samples diverged most in terms of the 'moderately isolated' group. Indeed, examination of the literature reveals the most variation in terms of the relative size of this population. Consequently, the 'moderately isolated' group may be the most likely to vary over time, with the measures used to determine the extent or reflect the composition of the populations surveyed. Within our two populations the distribution of isolation was similar, again highlighting the link with marital status. However, in this case it was the single, never married, who appeared to be most vulnerable. This may be an artefact of our measure as one of the variables is concerned with family contact. If the single have smaller families, this may explain this observation. This is clearly an area worthy of further investigation. The degree to which older people were engaged in a range of civic activities was broadly similar between the studies.

In relation to loneliness, our studies illustrate the two main approaches towards the empirical measurement of this phenomenon; self-report measures and the development of scales or aggregate measures (Wenger 1983). Self-report measures are simple to use, appear to be highly acceptable to research participants and ask directly about feelings of loneliness. However, their simplicity has been seen as a weakness, in that the question presumes a common understanding of the concept by study participants. Furthermore, loneliness may be seen as a 'stigmatizing' concept compromising the identity of individuals. Consequently, study participants may express a 'public' view and not admit to feelings of loneliness. An alternative approach to the measurement of loneliness has been the development of specific scales such as that devised by de Jong Gierveld (1987). However, all the scales demonstrate cultural specificity and rely upon measuring loneliness via indirect questions relating to direct social engagement. Hence they make theoretical assumptions about the definition and meaning of loneliness and the link between social engagement and loneliness. Holmen and Furukawa (2002) suggest that the self-report measures are more appropriate for use with older people, although there is clearly still scope for considering empirically the merits of the different approaches.

The two studies reported here produced differing levels of loneliness among the populations surveyed. However, the level of loneliness in deprived areas was similar to that reported by Bowling et al. (1991) in their study of older people in the London Borough of Hackney. Loneliness appears to be more pronounced among older people living in areas characterized by intense social deprivation than in other residential settings. At this stage we can only speculate about the characteristics of deprived areas that might be associated with higher levels of loneliness. In part, the higher levels of loneliness demonstrated in the deprived areas as compared with the Omnibus Survey may reflect the differing nature of the two populations. In particular, the two samples differ in the extent of widowhood among those participating in the studies. In the deprived areas sample rates of widowhood were about one-third higher than in the Omnibus Survey. Given that widowhood is a key independent risk factor for loneliness, this may, in part, account for the observed differences between our two samples. However, given the similarity of the levels of loneliness in the deprived areas study and those reported by Bowling et al. (1991), we might speculate that the differences between our two groups are more than the result of simple artefact. For example, such variation may be related to factors that inhibit the development and maintenance of stable social relationships within specific spatial locations. Despite the fact that most older people in deprived areas are long-term residents of their communities (79 per cent of respondents had lived in their neighbourhood for 20 years or more), high population turnover, fear of crime, and low levels of interpersonal trust might combine to reduce the intensity and quality of such relationships. This also raises questions about the degree to which older people who are lonely are surrounded by other people who are lonely. In this respect, one could argue that certain types of urban neighbourhood might represent pockets of loneliness – either by attracting people who are already lonely, or by engendering loneliness within older people under the influence of a range of neighbourhood characteristics. However, our two studies were consistent in linking loneliness with marital status and clearly highlighted the vulnerability of widowed elders to this experience. In both studies, marriage appeared to act as a factor that protects older people from feelings of loneliness.

Conclusion

The focus in the majority of studies of social exclusion and participation among older people are predominantly cross-sectional in nature. As such, our understanding of these aspects of later life are static and lacking in a biographical or lifecourse perspective. We suggest that there is a clear need to locate our understanding within a more dynamic framework, and to be able to compare and contrast the experience of social exclusion in later life with that experienced at other phases of the life cycle. This perspective would enable us to investigate three distinct types of perspectives upon social exclusion in later life: (a) as a continuation of patterns from earlier phases of life; (b) as a new experience; or (c) as the reduction from previous patterns. We can speculate that the factors associated with these differing types of loneliness and isolation may vary, and that potential interventions to ameliorate them may need to reflect this complexity. Longitudinal studies of loneliness and isolation, such as those undertaken by Holmen and Furukawa (2002), Wenger and Burholt (2004) and Tijhuis et al. (1999) offer a more robust method for identifying such typologies than cross-sectional studies and may offer insights into the nature and type of social interventions that might help combat this negative aspect of later life. Biographical and life review studies as well as case studies can also enhance our understanding of the dynamics of social engagement. However, given the limitations of our methods, our two datasets indicate the overall high levels of social engagement illustrated by contemporary elders and suggest that levels of social contact, isolation and loneliness have not changed dramatically in the post-war period, despite the numerous social changes manifest over this period.

Acknowledgements

We wish to acknowledge the contribution of a range of organizations to the research described in this chapter. Both studies were funded by the Economic and Social Research Council as part of its Growing Older Programme (award numbers L480254042 and L480254022). The Quality of Life Survey was also part-funded by grants held by Professor Ann Bowling (award number L480254043 – also part of the Growing Older Programme) and Professor Shah Ebrahim (Medical Research Council Health Services Research Collaboration). The deprived areas study received additional financial support from Help the Aged. In relation to the Quality of Life Survey, we are grateful to the Office for National Statistics (ONS) Omnibus Survey Unit for overseeing the fieldwork and preparing the dataset. Those who carried out the original analysis and collection of the data hold no responsibility for the further analysis and interpretation of them. Material from the ONS Omnibus Survey, made available through ONS, has been used with the permission of the Controller of The Stationery Office. Both datasets are held at the ESRC Data Archive at the University of Essex. We are indebted to our co-investigators, Professors John Bond, Ann Bowling, Paul Kingston and Chris Phillipson for their contributions to the projects upon which this chapter is based and to the researchers who worked on the projects: Dr Sasha Scambler and Allison E. Smith. Finally we would like to thank our interviewers, and we are especially grateful to all those older people who gave so freely of their time to participate in these studies.

Note

1 Both studies included a qualitative in-depth interview component which is not reported here for reasons of space. Semi-structured interviews were conducted with 130 people living in deprived areas (90 of whom had taken part in the first phase of the research), and 45 people from the national survey (all of whom were involved in the first stage of the study). Fieldwork for both studies was completed in 2001/2002.

8

Frailty, identity and the quality of later life

Kevin McKee, Murna Downs, Mary Gilhooly, Ken Gilhooly, Susan Tester and Fiona Wilson

Introduction

Within Western societies negative stereotypes of old age are common. Prevalent stereotypes are that most older people are: confused, resigned to decline, tired, slow, dependent (Unsworth et al. 2001). Stereotypes tend to restrict and guide people's thought processes, and researchers themselves are not free of stereotypical thinking. It is therefore unsurprising that dominant research paradigms in geriatrics and gerontology have sought to chart a map of decline in later life, and classify older people in terms of the problems that they face. Older people are described in terms of their 'functional impairment', 'functional performance', their level of 'dependency' or 'frailty' (Woodhouse et al. 1988; Jarrett et al. 1995; Rockwood et al. 1999). Given these deeply held representations of old age, it is no surprise that old age, as an identity, is something that people resist and perceive negatively – even older people themselves (Netz and Ben-Sira 1993).

The mental connection between ageing and a decline in physical health is so strong that similar symptoms presented by people of different ages may be interpreted differently. A sharp pain in the chest of a 25-year-old may be considered the result of indigestion or muscle strain, while pain in the chest of a 70-year-old is more likely to be interpreted as the signal of a myocardial infarction. A person of 30 falling over may be thought clumsy or drunk, while a fall in a 70-year-old is more likely to be attributed to frailty. These 'attributional biases' occur in both young and old age groups. Williamson and Fried (1996) found that 31 per cent of a sample of 230 community dwelling older people cited old age as the cause of difficulty in one or more tasks of daily living, with 20 per cent of the sample citing old age as the cause in two or more tasks.

Perceiving old age as a cause of physical disability can have serious psychological consequences. 'Old age' is stable (it does not go away) and global (affecting all aspects of life), and thus fulfils the criteria for a causative factor that is consistent with a hopelessness explanatory style (Abramson et al. 1989). Here we have a potential catalyst for the transition between the Third Age and the Fourth Age (Laslett 1991), that is, from someone living an active later life, to someone compromised by the challenges of age. This transition has been referred to as the Body Drop (McKee 1998). A Body Drop occurs when a sudden failure of functioning of the body is attributed to stable and global factors, such as ageing. The attribution leads to poor recovery from the failure, since the person believes that the cause of the failure is not remediable.

The Body Drop is fundamentally a transition in self-identity, through which an individual comes to think of himself or herself as someone who is no longer in an endless 'middle-youth' (Featherstone and Hepworth 1991), but as someone who is old. As Goffman (1963) argues, management of the body is central to a person's identity, and their ability to present a version of the self that is preferred rather than stigmatizing. As a person ages, one might expect the discrepancy between a 'subjective sense of inner youthfulness and an exterior process of biological ageing' (Turner 1995: 258), to create more psychological and behavioural demands. When a major failure of the body occurs, such as stroke, or a hip fracture from a fall, the psychological reserves of the person may be presented with a challenge that cannot, finally, be met. The result is an assimilation of the young 'inner' self by the old, malfunctioning external self.

Ageing, then, involves a transformation of the individual from a person who considers himself or herself as young and valued, to someone who sees himself or herself as frail and disabled, a move from a desired to an undesired self (Markus and Nurius 1986). As a respondent in a study by Fournier and Fine (1990: 340) expresses, 'Getting *old* means getting weaker. When you get old, you hate to have people see you in a weakened condition. It depresses you.' Interestingly, there is no consistent evidence that people get more dissatisfied with their body as they age. Indeed, some studies have shown the reverse – that older people report greater body satisfaction than young people (for example, Öberg and Tornstam 1999; Reboussin et al. 2000). Research does suggest, however, that an older person's body satisfaction relative to a younger person's is more related to body function than body appearance, and that body function is strongly related to well-being (Reboussin et al. 2000).

Self and identity in old age, along with being influenced by the body, can also be considered as a function of social interactions. This social psychological view of the self is most notably captured in Mead's (1934) symbolic interactionism. Here the self is viewed as being fundamentally a social structure, arising from, and developing within, social interactions and relationships in which symbols or meanings are shared. Viewing the experience of self in old age through this lens extends the gaze beyond the older person's body to the nature of their relationships and interactions with others. From this standpoint, the role of the other in supporting identity and self in older people becomes critical. Such a perspective requires that studies of self and quality of life (QoL) in old age include the person's social context and relationships.

There has been a long research tradition exploring QoL of older people in institutional settings which demonstrates the negative effect on identity and self of social structures in these settings (Townsend 1962). These settings are associated with social interactions that undermine identity and self, referred to by Kitwood (1997) as Malignant Social Psychology. To counteract this tendency Kitwood (1997) proposed a person-centred approach to care emphasizing the key role played by empathic and supportive relationships in promoting QoL (Brooker, forthcoming). What is less well known is how frailty, both physical and mental, and social interactions and relationships intersect to affect self and identity in these settings. Bruce and colleagues (2002) argue, on the basis of their longitudinal study, that those with the greatest mental and physical frailty receive the least opportunity for engagement in social interaction. Following the symbolic interactionist's line of argument, self and identity will be most threatened and least supported for those with the greatest physical and mental frailty.

Resisting frailty

Is there a possibility for an older person to resist the negative implications of frailty for their personal well-being? In recent decades, there has been a growth in theory that places ageing within a positive context. Rowe and Kahn's (1987) model of successful ageing, and Baltes and Baltes (1990) model of optimal ageing both examined the factors that promoted positive outcomes in late life. However, even in the more traditional models of late life ageing, there are indications that the link between frailty and well-being can be moderated. In activity theory, there is an emphasis on continuity through the life span, and a central tenet is that 'those who are able to remain socially active will be more likely to achieve a positive self-image, social integration and satisfaction with life' (Barrow 1992: 70). However, it is recognized in the theory that the forms of social activity that can be achieved will alter with advancing age. The challenge is for the older person to find forms of social activity that will enhance their well-being, and yet which will not be hindered by frailty (Brandtstadter and Renner 1990). For example, there is good evidence that reminiscence might benefit the psychological health of older people (Brooker and Duce 2000; Cully et al. 2001; Hsieh and Wang 2003). Reminiscence is usually considered as a general look back to days gone by, with one of the most accepted definitions put forward by Woods et al. (1992: 138): 'The vocal or silent recall of events in a person's life, either alone or with another person or group of people.' Within Erikson's life-span development model (Erikson et al. 1986), reminiscence plays a key role at the final stage of life, as a potential catalyst in resolving psychologically damaging regrets, and helping an older person achieve ego-integrity. Considering reminiscence from within an activity theory framework, as an older person becomes increasingly frail and the potential to engage in physically demanding social activities becomes compromised, replacing such activities with others that make few physical demands, such as reminiscence, could help the older person retain their social engagement, and also maintain levels of well-being. From within a symbolic interactionist framework, reminiscence could be a focus of interaction that will enhance an older person's identity and sense of self.

Researching frailty and identity in later life

In this part of the chapter we draw on findings from three research projects within the Growing Older Programme to explore aspects of self and identity in frail older age, including the impact of reminiscence on QoL, the role of relationships in maintaining sense of self, and ways in which older people resist mental frailty.

Study 1 Reminiscence and discontinuity of the self in frail older people

Between February 2000 and May 2002, a qualitative study was carried out to determine the impact of reminiscence activity on the QoL of older people. Data were collected via semi-structured interviews with older people in residential care, focus groups with care staff, older people in care, and their family carers (McKee et al. 2002).

The key themes that emerged from the analyses of the focus group transcripts were found to operate at three different levels. Level one themes demonstrated that sharing past and present lives through talk was a central aspect of building relationships between residents and between residents and care staff. At the second level, everyday talk concerning the past appeared to offer intergenerational benefits. Older people were central to the transmission and preservation of family folklore, and this activity helped to preserve the identity of the older person as well as providing them with a significant role within the family context. At the third level, while past and present talk helped people to share lives and feel valued, there were tensions that could impede this process. Staff recognize that talking meaningfully about the past and present can be distressing for an older person, and that staff may not have the skills or time to address sensitive interactions competently. An organizational commitment to value social care and equip staff to focus on listening and talking as more than 'just chatting' could enhance interactions and facilitate a relationship-centred focus of care.

Importantly, older people often expressed a sense of loss, for example, of friends and relations, of functional or cognitive ability, or of their home. This was related to an experience of discontinuity in their personal identity and from the present world, a world to which they felt they did not belong. Sensory or memory loss, for example, could inhibit social and interpersonal interaction. As one family carer explained:

> I think mother is aware that she's actually losing it a bit, and I think she feels embarrassed getting into a conversation with people she doesn't know, because (a) as you say, she doesn't know this area, but (b) she realizes that she's getting a bit confused. But she's been sitting at a table with three other ladies since September and she still can't remember their names.

While relatives provided opportunities for intergenerational reminiscence, carers or younger family seemed unable to 'connect' and provide the comradeship and familiarity of the past that could be provided by peers. The loss of same-aged friends was therefore acutely felt.

A second theme around discontinuity focused on a gap between past and present. Older people expressed the feeling that the present was not *their* world, but a hostile and lonely place. This was reflected in the continual comparison between past and present, in which the past was always presented more favourably than the present, as this quote from on older male resident demonstrates:

> I wouldn't like to relive my life again, not in this world. The world's all right but it's the people that live in it – villains and vicious people. They'll do anything for money now – murder, tie pensioners up.

For some, the hostile present precipitated a return to the past, as this daughter indicated was the case for her father:

> If he said for some reason or another he wanted to go home, he wasn't talking about where we were living, he wasn't talking about where I'd moved him from where they'd lived for 60 years, he was talking about his childhood as a little boy. He wanted to go back to where he was a little boy.

A third theme of discontinuity related to being cut off or displaced. Being 'cut off' as a result of frailty and a loss of friends gave a sense of discontinuity that triggered reminiscence, as expressed by a care staff member:

> I do I think they love it [reminiscence]. They don't get out that often, so they're cut off from the world kind of thing, but their world that they remember is the past, so therefore that's what they enjoy.

Older participants frequently expressed feelings of displacement, perhaps particularly pertinent in a generation of older people with war experiences. One male resident noted:

> There's many a time – well, most nights, I'll sit out on the front for ten minutes and thought about running away. I felt I was in a remand home. I hate feeling locked in, and I don't know, I suppose there are other people in the same boat . . . but it is me that's locked in.

Carers, however, felt that a reciprocal sharing of lives and the building of relationships using both past and present talk, could mediate or overcome feelings of discontinuity.

This piece of research suggests that reminiscence can be a powerful influence on identity maintenance for older people. Frail older people can offer up a past, preferred identity that has significance and richness, in contrast perhaps to their current identity that offers them little status. Through transmitting family narratives to children and grandchildren, an older person can again demonstrate the significance of events that they enacted in their past lives, and occupy a key family role. However, there is a danger that, through its concentration on the past, reminiscence locates older people in the past, only. Having someone listen to older people's concerns about their present lives might be more meaningful to them than conversations about the past, and care staff and family members should be encouraged to address older people's feelings of discontinuities in the self and from the present world. Activities encouraging meaningful linkage of the past with the present are essential in order to provide a sense of continuity to an older person's lifecourse, and address feelings of discontinuity in identity commonly expressed by participants.

Study 2 The role of relationships in maintaining a sense of self

The second study also took a qualitative approach to exploring perceptions of QoL of frail older people following a move to a care home (Tester et al. 2003). The study aimed to include older people with all types of physical and/or mental disabilities or conditions. Data were collected using focus groups, 24-hour observation in four care home settings, and observation and interviews with 52 residents in care homes for older people. After transition to institutional care, frail older people may experience continuities and discontinuities in maintaining their identity. Four key inter-related areas were identified as components of QoL: (1) sense of self; (2) the care environment; (3) relationships; and (4) activities. We focus here on the project's findings on the role of personal relationships in maintaining a sense of self.

Although moving into a care home entailed the loss of familiar company for some participants, it also provided a potential opportunity for forming new relationships. Communication, both verbal and non-verbal, is essential in the development and maintenance of relationships with other residents. For people with sensory and/or cognitive impairments, non-verbal communication can convey feelings and meanings important in the development of relationships (Hubbard et al. 2002). However, there were practical and attitudinal barriers to communication among residents. The loss or non-use of hearing aids was a common practical barrier to conversation.

Attitudes to others among the group of frail older people living together ranged from hostility and indifference to sympathy and friendship. Indifference to other residents was common as they were seen as irrelevant, for example:

> Don't bother with them. I don't bother with that. They don't bother me. (Denis Samuels)[1]

> Well, it doesn't really matter to me – just miss them out. (Gordon Miller)

> They're all right, they're only residents. (Christina Strong)

Hostility was seen in the reactions of some residents to others' behaviour. They distanced themselves from those labelled as 'mental', for example, by taking over particular lounges to avoid those so labelled, thus projecting their 'self' as not 'mental' (Hubbard et al. 2003). Such findings show that residents did have a sense of self in relation to others and could take on the role of others to interpret, make meaning of and react to their behaviour (Hubbard et al. 2002).

In spite of such hostility, distancing and indifference, some participants did develop relationships with other residents, showing friendship and friendliness towards them. The women were more likely than the men to present themselves as generally friendly. Some had established friendly relationships, for example, regularly sitting together in a particular lounge. However, having a special friend among the other residents was rare. Some had developed a friendship through knowing each other earlier in their lives, or through a shared experience such as both having Parkinson's disease, or being smokers. For some women participants, having a friend could be a form of protection from a potentially harmful environment. For example, Amy Logan, who expressed anger about the home and the way the staff treated her, said that she and her friend were 'very quiet . . . we just sit there and listen to what's going on'.

There was some evidence that the level of involvement of relatives in participants' lives could make a difference to their self-confidence and ability to form relationships with people in the care home. Continuity of family life, with spouses, children and other relatives was also important in maintaining a sense of self. Married life was important to QoL, whether or not the spouse was still alive, and provided a store of memories and a sense of identity. The involvement of children and grandchildren through visits, gifts and services provided, brought interest to participants' lives and gave them a sense of being part of a family. In the case of Doreen McCall, whose sons and daughters living nearby visited daily, and that of Maureen Stone, whose husband and daughter took turns to visit most days, living in an institution did not act as a barrier to the resident's inclusion in family life. These women both conveyed a strong sense of themselves and their success in forming friendships.

Relationships with spouses, parents and siblings who may no longer be alive appeared to be salient to the present QoL of people with dementia. Mills and Coleman (1994) show that people with dementia are able to recall parts of their past biographies. Thus, it is important to offer opportunities to talk about their life history and to support people in retaining a sense of self by building on the strengths of emotional memories of the self (Mills 1997).

These findings exemplify ways in which frail older people living in care homes were able to maintain a sense of self through interaction and relationships with others in the home, through developing new friendships, and through continuity of close emotional ties with spouses and family members and maintaining a sense of being part of a family. Consistent with the symbolic interactionist perspective the study found that care workers have an important role in supporting residents' interaction and communication and their ability to maintain and develop relationships, thus enhancing their QoL and sense of self.

Study 3 Resisting mental frailty in old age

Although physical frailty is certainly unwelcome, it is mental frailty that is most feared by older people (Gilhooly et al. 1986). Dementia and cognitive failure strike at our very 'personhood', our self-identity (Aronson and Lipkowitz 1981; Kastenbaum 1988; Chiverton and Caine 1989). The literature on 'personhood', although varied in terms of definitions, generally suggests that characteristics such as the ability to think rationally, sensible communications, and independent goal-directed activities are important to personhood. When an individual ceases to be able to perform these functions, they may cease to be 'persons' and may even be candidates for 'social death' (Sweeting and Gilhooly 1992).

Gilhooly and her colleagues examined the extent to which older people believe it is possible to resist mental frailty and what, if anything, older people do to prevent cognitive decline (K. Gilhooly et al. 2003; M. Gilhooly et al. 2002b, 2003). Although there is much folklore associated with the 'use it or lose it' hypothesis in relation to brain ageing, there is relatively little research on the extent to which engaging in mental, social or physical activity might delay or prevent cognitive decline and dementia. Moreover, what research exists on this issue is contradictory. While there are several studies suggesting that there are positive relationships between participation in cognitively stimulating activities and cognitive ability (Gold et al. 1995; Ball et al. 2002) and even reduced risk of Alzheimer's disease (Wilson et al 2002), there are also a number of studies which have found that age-related declines in cognitive functioning are not ameliorated by engagement in activities (Hambrick et al. 1999; Salthouse et al. 2002).

Study participants were asked what three things contribute to good mental functioning in old age. Also examined were frequencies of physical, mental and social behaviours that might maintain good cognitive functioning. Each item was given a score of 'numbers of days per year' in which the activity was undertaken. Composite scores were created for the three main categories of activity (Glass et al. 1999). The following activities were considered: (1) mental activities – read newspapers, read books, play cards, play chess, do crosswords, write letters, work with computer, listen to music, sew, knit, bingo; (2) physical activities – swimming, dancing, keep fit, golfing, fishing, gardening, do-it-yourself, walking, bowling; (3) social activities – see friends, see relatives, social club, attend meeting, voluntary work, attend religious service. Study participants were also asked to rate their QoL.

What are the attitudes and beliefs of older people in relation to what can be done to prevent cognitive decline in old age?

In response to the question about three things which could be done to maintain good cognitive functioning in old age, many respondents merely noted 'having an interest/keeping interested', keeping busy/keeping active, followed by doing crosswords/puzzles. Responses became more specific for second and third choices. The pattern changed somewhat, with socializing with family and friends noted more frequently. Also, the importance of physical activity for maintaining good cognitive functioning in old age increased in salience by the time respondents were naming their second and third choices of activities. Church and volunteer work also became more prominent by the third response, as did the view that 'contentment' or general attitude to life could be important. Under 'miscellaneous' were coded single responses such as money and betting. Thus, although somewhat vague as to exactly what could be done to prevent mental frailty in old age, most study participants were of the view that something could be done. Keeping active and busy was viewed as important, as was engaging in activities that required mental work. Keeping physically active was noted, but did not emerge as something which most of the respondents thought would have a major impact on cognitive functioning.

To what extent do older adults deliberately engage in physical and mental activities to prevent cognitive decline?

Some 60 per cent of the study participants indicated deliberately undertaking activities aimed at maintaining good cognitive functioning. The activities noted were classified as gentle and vigorous physical activity, passive mental activity, mental activity requiring planning, and passive and involved social activities. The highest proportion of activities noted was classified as mental activity requiring planning (for example, crosswords) (70 per cent), followed by passive mental activities (for example, reading) (47 per cent). Passive social activity was mentioned by 15 per cent of those deliberately undertaking activities with the purpose of maintaining good cognitive functioning. Slightly fewer than 8 per cent of the sample mentioned activities classified as 'involved social activity'. Some 17 per cent of the sample said they undertook gentle physical activity to maintain good cognitive functioning in old age, with 16 per cent indicating that they engaged in what they viewed as vigorous physical activity. These figures suggest little belief in a strong mind–body relationship. On the other hand, it may be that, due to their advanced age, study participants found it more difficult to engage in physical activities.

To what extent was engagement in physical, mental and social activities associated with cognitive functioning?

There were three significant correlations between mental activities (composite scores) and three of the psychometric tests used to assess current cognitive functioning, namely, the WAIS matrix reasoning, digit substitution scales, and the category fluency test. There were no significant associations between social activities and physical activities and performance on the psychometric tests.

To what extent was engagement in physical, mental and social activities and cognitive functioning associated with quality of life?

Of special interest to this chapter were the findings on the relationships between activity levels and reported QoL. On the whole, ratings of levels of social and physical activity, though significant, were not highly correlated with ratings of QoL. Interestingly, ratings of mental activities were not correlated with reported QoL at all. Furthermore, QoL ratings were not highly correlated with measures of cognitive functioning, with the exception of 'real-world' problem solving. However, self-rated assessments of cognitive functioning were associated with ratings of QoL, with those rating themselves as functioning at higher levels of cognitive functioning also rating their QoL as higher.

In summary, participants in this study indicated a general belief that 'keeping active' was important for good cognitive functioning in old age, with 60 per cent indicating that they engaged in some activity with the aim of resisting cognitive decline. The link between estimated volume of mental activity engaged in over the year and certain aspects of actual cognitive functioning supports the 'use it or lose it' notion of ways to resist cognitive decline in old age. However, it was interesting that there was no association between engagement in social or physical activities and cognitive functioning. There was, as in other studies of a cross-sectional nature, also no way of disentangling cause and effect. Did engagement in mental activity prevent decline, or were those who were functioning at higher levels of cognitive abilities more likely to engage in mental activities?

It was somewhat surprising to find that participation in social activities was not associated with perceived QoL, given the volume of literature indicating that engagement with family and friends is important to happiness (Myers 2000). It may, of course, be that the measures of QoL in this study placed too much emphasis on health or other factors that swamped the relationships between activities and QoL. The very advanced age of the sample, combined with the fact that half were selected to be 'unhealthy', may also account for the dominance of current health and morbidity history as predictors of QoL, compared to mental, social and physical activities.

What was, however, interesting was that perceived (and self-rated) cognitive functioning was associated with perceived QoL. It should, perhaps, not be surprising that those who report poor, or declining, cognitive functioning also report poorer QoL. There is a growing body of literature suggesting that the opportunity to take part in valued activities across the life span contributes to well-being above and beyond the effects of 'having' various material, personal and social resources (Canter and Sanderson 1999). Declining cognitive functioning is likely to be perceived as negatively impacting on one's ability to take part in valued activities, as well as on one's pursuit of and progress towards goals. In addition, real or perceived decline in mental functioning is likely to be associated with perceptions of personal control. There is a large literature suggesting that perceptions of personal control are important for well-being (Peterson 1999).

Conclusion

The three projects discussed above all used inclusive methods, but took varying approaches to different groups of frail older people. There were, however, common issues that emerged from the findings. The themes of discontinuity and loss linked the projects in various ways. Frail participants experienced discontinuity in their personal identity through loss of their home, loss of friends and familiar company, decline in physical health or cognitive functioning, feeling cut off in the present world, or being indifferent to fellow residents.

To counter such discontinuities, identity could be maintained in ways that focused on positive continuities such as having a significant role in the family, keeping active and sustaining cognitive functioning. Communication played a key role in maintaining identity, through building and sustaining relationships and friendships; through reminiscence and opportunities to talk about life histories; and through participation in meaningful activities. It was through interaction and communication that participants were able to keep a sense of self in relation to others. The project's findings identified ways in which care staff and family carers can enhance communication and relationships, listen to older people's concerns about the present, and promote the identity and QoL of frail older people in different settings and circumstances.

Acknowledgements

Mary and Ken Gilhooly would like to note that Ms Dominique Harvey and Ms Allison Murray deserve a special acknowledgement for their contribution to their GO project as research assistants. Mrs Margaret Lothian participated in data collection on the 'lay concepts' component of the study, as did Susan Caldwell, Eileen McDonach and Karen Dunleavy.

Murna Downs and Susan Tester would like to acknowledge the significant contributions of the other members of the project team, Gill Hubbard, Charlotte MacDonald and Joan Murphy. We are grateful to all the participants, staff and managers of the homes included in the study. We also gratefully acknowledge the advice and contributions of the project advisory group, colleagues, research postgraduates, and GO programme participants.

Kevin McKee and Fiona Wilson would like to acknowledge their co-workers on the Economic and Social Research Council (Award No.: L480254031) project 'Evaluating the impact of reminiscence on the QoL of older people', part of the GO programme: Gillie Bolton, Man Cheung Chung, Helen Elford, Fiona Goudie, Sharron Hinchliff and Cindy Mitchell.

Note

1   Pseudonyms are used for all participants.

9

Identity, meaning and social support

Christopher McKevitt, John Baldock, Jan Hadlow,
Jo Moriarty and Jabeer Butt

Introduction

This chapter uses findings from three studies which were part of the Growing Older programme to illuminate the ways in which older people use social support services. Its key argument is that the use of care services is mediated through a more important activity: the maintenance and reconstruction of identities and social relationships made necessary by increased dependence on help from others. The first study was of 41 people aged between 60 and 90 who had returned home from hospital after surviving a stroke. The second was of 38 people over 75, living on their own who had recently experienced a decline in their health that had left them unable to leave home without assistance. The third was of 203 people, of whom the majority were from a minority ethnic group. Although not everyone in this sample had recently undergone a severe illness, three-quarters reported that they had a long-standing illness or disability and, of these, over 80 per cent felt that it affected their everyday lives.

Each study included many people in their eighties and some well over 90. These people are part of a demographic phenomenon sometimes known as the 'longevity revolution', which describes the growing numbers of people surviving into great old age. One consequence of this success is to reinforce professional and medical models of old age. Such models are not without foundation or evidence of success but they need to be mediated in practice through an understanding of how older people and their families respond to the help they receive. The social gerontology literature shows how in later life, and particularly with the onset of disabilities, people engage in 'identity work' in order to readjust to new circumstances and to maintain a sense of self-worth (Kaufman 1986; Thompson et al. 1990). This identity work does not focus solely on medical problems or practical care needs, but on rebuilding self-esteem and a sense of self consistent with the revised social and family circumstances that come with increased disability and new needs for help. In this context 'rational' or 'practical' responses can take second place to those that are more personally appropriate to a person's identity project. These three studies illustrate that there are imperatives requiring older people to integrate medical and social care with a sustaining self-image and with acceptable social and family relationships. Roy Porter's classic study points out how these tensions between the personal, the social and the technical are inherent in the Western conception of medicine and health:

> The West has evolved a culture preoccupied with the self, with the individual and his or her identity ... whereas most traditional healing systems have sought to understand the relations of the sick person to the wider cosmos and to make readjustments between the individual and the world, or society and the world, the western medical tradition explains sickness principally in terms of the body itself – its own cosmos. (Porter 1997: 6)

The stroke study

The first study, *An Anthropological Investigation of Lay and Professional Meanings of Quality of Life*, examined the concept of quality of life (QoL) and its measurement in the context of a stroke and stroke care. It aimed to contribute to a sociological understanding of the epistemological basis of the concept of QoL and the ramifications of its application. Here we draw on material collected during interviews with stroke patients aged 60 and over.

Two-stage interviews were conducted; the first held once patients had been given a discharge date from hospital and the second, three months later. Forty one people participated in first interviews, with 33 subsequently participating in a second interview. Interviewees' ages ranged from 61–90. Six were Black Caribbean or African with the remainder being white British or other European; 21 were men.

The longer-term consequences of a stroke can include reduced ability to use limbs, leading to problems of mobility, self-care, and other activities, impaired cognitive function, communication and memory; problems with sight; and psychological effects, including mood disorders and depression. It has been estimated that 35 per cent of those with a stroke who survive beyond one year are significantly disabled and need help with basic daily tasks (Stephen and Raftery 1994). However, this may be an underestimation since the measures used to quantify disability may not adequately reflect people's ability to carry out activities that they consider important. Certainly, study participants who were classified as 'functionally independent' commonly identified consequences of stroke that hindered their ability to lead their life as they would choose.

Services for stroke survivors in the community may include clinic, community or home-based rehabilitation therapies, access to supported discharge schemes, and a range of local authority statutory services (such as home care, meals on wheels, or respite care) as well as those provided by voluntary sector organizations. Overwhelmingly, people primarily rely on family members to provide assistance and their use of formal services is secondary (Anderson 1988). For example, three months after the onset of stroke among people living in the community, 10 per cent of people on the South London Stroke Register had used the meals on wheels service, 27 per cent home care, and 7 per cent had attended a day centre. These proportions declined one year after stroke, except in the case of day centre use, where it had slightly increased (McKevitt et al. 2003).

Sources of social support

For participants in this study, social support came primarily from family (spouse/partner, children, siblings, other kin) and, to a lesser extent, friends. In this way providing and receiving support were bound up with long-standing affective relationships in which love, responsibility and duty underpinned caring and being cared for. Mrs M returned home after her stroke without physical disabilities but some confusion and fatigue. She lived alone but was cared for by her daughter, brother, and other family members. Her daughter commented:

> I mean, we're all very close, yeah, it's always been like that, so there's no difference really, relying on me probably a bit more, that's changed, but apart from that, nothing's changed, has it?

There was recognition that adult children 'have their own lives' and that assistance should not disrupt that. At the same time expectations about the extent of care that could be given were not completely clear and had to be negotiated. This was made especially apparent during an interview in which the subject of respite care was broached. Mrs J reminded her husband that a social worker had talked to her about having a rest from caring:

Mrs J: So . . . [the] first thing she said to me was, you know, about getting away for a break, she said, 'I thought there was something, you know, you was gonna do something', and I said, 'Well, not at the moment we haven't', she said I should try and get away.

Mr J: Yeah, but . . . I'm not in a fit state to get out of the house yet, let alone go for holidays.

Mrs J: But she's also thinking of me getting a, you know, which, erm . . .

This situation was extreme but exemplifies the dilemmas that families can face. Discharged from hospital to a nursing home, Mrs K had visits from siblings and spent weekends with her married son. She was distressed that her daughter had not been to see her for four months and blamed herself for asking her daughter to look after her at home:

She said no I don't blame her, cos I had the same life with my Mum, you see, I looked after her, so I don't blame her. Yeah, I think that's why she's not been back to see me . . . might not be that, but I've got a feeling it is.

Friends and neighbours were also important but here expectations about the boundaries of what might be legitimate were clearer. For example, Mr D's main source of support was his long-term partner who lived some distance away but spent every day with him. During the interview, they discussed frankly the need for his partner to have 'a little break'. They applied to a voluntary organization for assistance:

Cos there's nobody else, you see . . . I went away on holiday in February, but one of our friends took over . . . but there's very few we can call on. I mean, you know, they've all got their own lives, they're busy, some are working, you know.

Participants also described using other support strategies, including keeping in touch with family and friends by telephone, using alarms for emergencies, and investigating the use of technology to improve mobility and visual ability.

Many participants used, or had used, services such as supported discharge schemes, home care services and meals on wheels. Although some were satisfied, common complaints recurred. Typically, meals on wheels were criticized for being expensive and unpalatable. Those who rejected the service explained it in terms of preferring to make their own choice:

I don't want them to dictate to me what I eat . . . I think it's about three quid, isn't it? Right, I can go over the road and buy stuff. I mean, if I want chips, I'll have chips. If I want avocado, I have avocado. I have what I want.

Home help services were criticized for a range of reasons, including inadequate or too infrequent visits and high staff turnover ('They were all, they were all, they were all just anxious to get in and out.').

Service use and identity management

Apart from complaints about quality, there were other important reasons behind people's preference not to have these services. One explanation related to the importance attached to independence. For Mr G, physical, economic and social independence were intertwined:

> I wouldn't like to be a burden on anybody, you know. I mean, we've never had a home help or anything like that . . . not yet, anyway . . . that's our choice, you know. We're not on social or anything like that. That's why I like to keep myself independent. I mean, if such a time as I've got to go on social then I will, you know. But at the moment we get enough money to keep ourselves going, you know, so we're independent from the state.

Another related to notions of family. Notwithstanding the ambiguities surrounding the limits of what is legitimate to ask for and receive, some accounts suggested participants' preferences for support related to distinctions between domestic and outside realms, the private from the public. An extreme example was provided by Mr T who had rejected going to a day care centre because he did not want to mix with strangers or be taken to the centre by strangers. Although he had used a personal care service initially, this was stopped as he regained some mobility. Similarly, his family rejected home care because they were not happy to have strangers in the house.

Stroke and identity

A number of studies investigating the impact of stroke on individuals' sense of identity have drawn on the theories mentioned in the introduction to this chapter that chronic illness creates a biographical disruption, disordering the affected individual's own sense of identity and creating the need to reconstruct identity and biography (Grant 1996; Kaufman 1998; Eaves 2000; Ellis-Hill et al. 2000). However, this position has been challenged in a study reporting that few participants described stroke as traumatic or leading to catastrophic changes in their life or sense of self which argued that being older and previous experiences of illness and hardship were factors that mediated any potential assault on identity (Pound et al. 1998). The suggestion that stroke and its consequences are not regarded as catastrophic has itself been subsequently disputed (Dowswell et al. 2000; Hart 2001).

In this study stroke did appear to disturb some participants' sense of self. One participant spoke poignantly about feeling she had become like a baby now that she needed to be looked after and was trying to relearn how to carry out tasks. Some couples experienced role reversal. Women, used to looking after their family and husband, now had to accept being looked after. A man who had cared for his disabled wife was left more disabled than her and their caring roles were inverted. Commonly, people related their disabilities to their sense of self because they prevented them from carrying out activities that were important to them, that defined who they were. Mr M, who lived alone, summed it up:

> Well, I'm . . . see, I'm not one for being on my own, the word is gregarious, I think. You know, mixing with people, being where there's a lot of people, feeling like one of the pack, so to speak. Yeah, that's, that's what I miss, is the camaraderie of people round you, you see that's what I miss.

However, the perceived magnitude of the impact of stroke that participants reported ranged across the spectrum, from being described as an 'annoyance' to being so devastating that one man reported considering suicide. Such evaluations did not correlate directly with observable levels of disability but rather were made with reference to a range of factors. Some referred to their own personality, explaining they were 'phlegmatic' or accepting when faced with adversity. Commonly, people reported that what cannot be changed or undone simply has to be accepted. Comparisons, with peers or upwards or downwards to those more or less fortunate, were also made. Other adverse life events were cited to help explain individual responses. Some also invoked their own life biography and notions of ageing, including ideas about a natural decline, to suggest that the stroke and its consequences had to be seen within that context. Finally, some introduced their own religious beliefs and hopes both to explain the reasons for their misfortune and to speak about death.

Becoming housebound through disability

The second study, *How Older People Adapt their Lives and their Selves to the Experience of Becoming Housebound*, was deliberately focused on the tensions between the need for social and medical care and the management of identity. We chose to study people aged 75 and over living on their own who had recently become unable to go out without assistance. The literature suggests that a key turning point in old age comes when illness or disability makes one housebound, that is, unable to go out without the help of others. This shift to dependence is particularly acute if one is living alone; many of the things one takes for granted – shopping, driving or using public transport, visiting friends, helping others, going to the doctor – become more complicated and dependent on the help of others. Much of the autonomy that defines the self is compromised and identity and relationships with others have to be re-negotiated.

The sample of 29 women and 9 men were interviewed twice in their own homes over a period of six months. The questionnaire was relatively open-ended and included validated measures such as the *Barthel Index* (Granger 1979) and the *General Health Questionnaire* (Goldberg 1978; Goldberg and Williams 1988). The project also used two scales developed by Coleman and colleagues for the Southampton Ageing Project (Coleman 1984; Coleman et al. 1993). The *Self-Esteem Scale* seeks to understand the sources of people's self-esteem and to measure broadly how strong it is and the *Life Course Interview* assesses continuities and discontinuities in people's sense of self.

Effects on self-esteem

The sample demonstrated markedly lower levels of self-esteem compared to those in the Southampton random sample, which included people at all levels of disability. However, their scores usually improved between the first and second interviews. For 21 people self-esteem appeared to rise over the six months, in only seven cases did the score fall and in only two instances was the fall substantial. Explanations were sought by examining the cases individually, starting with those showing the greatest gain in self-esteem. The findings are complex but a clear pattern emerged. Self-esteem remained high where there was strong family support or where the older person attributed it to 'inner resources' such as religious faith, a sense of humour or long-established ability to cope. It was more likely to be low and remain low where these reasons were not mentioned. In this sample, only three people showed distinct improvements in their physical health so recovery in health did not play a clear role in improving self-esteem. The most common reason for an increase was some intervention of 'others' in the sample's lives; starting to attend a day centre or increasing the days of attendance, making new friends, and starting to use or getting on better with a home help or personal carer. In most cases, these sources had not been mentioned or foreseen at the first inter-view. Day centres, home helps and personal carers, had often been positively resisted.

Perceptions of ability, disability and needs

A wish to be seen as a self-defining person was evident throughout. People were slow to mention their disabilities (things they could not do). They attributed their coping, or occasionally failure to cope, to 'the sort of person I am', that is, to personal strengths and weaknesses, less often than to outside causes. When talking about their lives, people talked most about feelings, relationships and self-images. These categories are different from those used by professionals who are likely to be assessing coping ability and where a need for support can be met by the available help and services. We identified a difference between 'self-talk' (feelings, relationships and selves) and 'needs talk' (resources, abilities and disabilities). Respondents largely used the first sort and focused on the continuities and improvements in their lives and relationships. The 'needs talk' of professionals is likely to focus more often on negative change and loss of continuity. This dichotomy was apparent in a comment from Mrs A about her GP: 'We get on, but he has a deathbed manner. I accuse him of ageism.'

Nearly half of the sample had rejected offers of services at one time or another and explained these refusals less in terms of a lack of needs but rather because they found the offers inconsistent with their images of self:

> You have to have a home help (carer) but nothing else. I refused and manage as best I can to get in and out of bed.

> They wanted me to have a home help as well as a carer to help me get dressed. Well, dressing was my real problem so I had the carer for three weeks then decided I could dress myself.

> They spent most of their time telling me what they would do for me – not what I needed or wanted.

Even where other evidence showed that respondents were receiving help from social services or family members, this might not be mentioned when they were invited to give accounts of their daily and weekly routines. On some occasions respondents would only confirm they were getting assistance from others when they were prompted to check that the unmentioned help was indeed being received. In particular, although 15 of the 38 respondents had received a community care assessment, no-one mentioned this until they were asked directly. This pattern appeared to be related to ways in which people perceived their abilities and problems. Particular medical conditions were mostly described early on, although some people suppressed very serious medical problems. However, people were much less likely to state explicitly the everyday things that their medical conditions meant they could not do. They talked of feelings and relationships and much less of practicalities.

The discrepancy between the 'official' and 'private' accounts of our respondents' lives presents a problem of explanation to which we can only suggest a solution based on the accounts of identity work in the literature. A closed questionnaire that focused specifically on needs and services might have quickly ascertained what these were. However, the point of the open-ended approach of this research, which asked people to describe their lives in their own terms with little prompting, was to understand their perceptions of the order of their lives. The external provider view of dependent older people's lives is one that highlights change, urgency and pattern. The older person's view, in contrast, is one of continuity, delay and no apparent pattern. There is a very sharp dichotomy between the long, slow days of a frail older person and the fast, active, time-pressured existence of a care worker. One analogy might be the contrast between the experience among airport users of sitting around and waiting compared with the perspectives of airport workers of vigorous activity, tight timetables and crisis management. In this world, the visits of home helps or the much more occasional ministrations of GPs, nurses and social workers, while welcome, were relatively unimportant in the overall experience of things. Feelings, ill health and pain, and both the good and bad of family and friends are much more significant features of life than the input of service providers. To switch to another crude analogy, professionals and other service providers are often viewed rather as a diner sees a waiter in an overcrowded restaurant; difficult to contact and influence, often distracted, slow and forgetful, and producing a rather unsatisfactory product when they eventually do deliver the meal. The waiter's perspective is surely different; of ceaseless activity and continuous interaction with customers.

Another explanation of the sample's apparent tendency to ignore or even deny their health and social needs could be their resistance to conventional images of old age. Older people do not necessarily have an enlightened or accepting approach to old age. Respondents in this study shared many of the more negative conceptions and images of ageing. Indeed, with few exceptions, they perceived very old age in terms of debility and senility. After completing the interviews, many respondents advised the researcher 'not to get old'. Services were generally seen as signposts along the downward path of ageing. There was also a tendency to define services as for people worse off than themselves:

The SS [i.e all public welfare help] are for people that cannot get around. I would rather not depend on them. Social services are for people who don't mind sitting on their bottoms and letting others do it.

I refused to go into residential care when it was offered, as you really have to be beyond doing anything for yourself.

I wouldn't go into a home unless I was unconscious or mental.

In a similar vein, refusing services was seen as a way of defining oneself as independent, or at least less dependent. However, this stance can be undermined by events and the pressure from others to accept help, particularly from one's family. There is for some an element of capitulation in the ultimate acceptance of needs:

I wanted to help myself, not sit and watch someone else do it.

I want to remain autonomous and independent . . . even having a home carer would inhibit my freedom to choose what I want to do without, at least, having to explain myself.

Most of the sample described ways in which they saw themselves on a downward trajectory. They described the fears that came from their current dependencies and greater fears of what they felt the future could bring. Many saw the main defence against the downward trend as their own feelings and attitudes to their disabilities of old age. Problems could be fought and transcended or they could be accepted but ignored as far as possible. In both cases, the dominant view was that mental attitude, rather than physical reality, was important. To use a service was seen as an admission of losing a battle. Others chose to accept a service for convenience but then did not want to dwell on it. Both strategies depended on resilience and alertness and very often also on humour:

I have hope even though the doctor doesn't encourage this . . . I'm going to get better and make the most of it. I'm going nowhere, if anything is going to happen it is going to happen here.

I have had to pull my socks up. My mind is very energetic. If my body doesn't want to do it, I make myself. When other people are down, I am up.

Quality of life and social support among people from different ethnic groups

The final study, *Quality of Life and Social Support among People from Different Ethnic Groups*, was developed in response to the increasing realization that while the United Kingdom, in common with the majority of societies in the developed world, has become increasing ethnically diverse, this is rarely reflected in published studies examining QoL (Smith 2000; Walker and Martimo 2000).

Instead, prevalent images of older people from minority ethnic groups often portray negative stereotypes (Blakemore and Boneham 1994). The exception to this largely pessimistic depiction is social support, which ironically represents a further stereotype whereby all people from minority ethnic groups are perceived as having access to extended families (Katbamna et al. 1998; Social Services Inspectorate 1998; Ahmad 2000). In this context, the growing literature on intersectionality (Calasanti 1996; Dressel et al. 1998; McMullin 2000) is especially useful. It demonstrates that, although some groups are more privileged than others in their experience of ageing, few people are privileged on all dimensions (Calasanti 2004). This is clearly demonstrated in existing studies based on ethnically diverse samples. Here, disadvantages in aspects such as income and health may be counterbalanced by advantages in others, such as social support (Nazroo et al. 2003) or having a meaningful role (Tsang et al. 2004). Furthermore, individuals continue to use different strategies to pursue satisfying lives (Afshar et al. 2002; Wray 2004).

The sample's experiences of different sources and types of social support is discussed elsewhere (Moriarty and Butt 2004). Here the focus is on how participants used it to give purpose and meaning to their lives. While support from family was generally seen as preferable to support from health and social care services, it was more common for these services not to have been offered than to have been rejected. Overall, participants from minority ethnic groups, despite associating ageing with disability and illness, also emphasized that the process had its positive aspects.

Some 203 interviews took place with people living in different parts of England and Scotland. The mean age of the sample was 69, with the youngest participant being 55 and the oldest 100. The numbers of men and women were almost equal. Participants' ethnicity reflected the historical patterns of immigration to the UK during the 1960s and 1970s, with over half the sample consisting of Black Caribbeans (n = 55) and Asian Indians (n = 55). Some 13 participants defined themselves as Asian Pakistani and the remainder consisted of Chinese people (n = 11), Black Africans (n = 7), Asian Bangladeshis (n = 5) and people from other ethnic groups or of mixed heritage (n = 17). Just under a fifth of participants were white (n = 38).

Service use and identity management

Policy decisions about the forms of support required by older people must be informed by an understanding of the boundaries between the 'public' world of the community and the 'private' sphere of the individual and the family (Finch 1989; Biggs 1993). When asked 'if people are no longer able to look after themselves in old age, whose responsibility should it be to provide support for them?', participants expressed considerable consensus about the need for flexible partnerships between the family, the state and individuals:

> Support should come from the children but my children [live far] away from me. It is not possible for them . . . [The responsibility is] is that of social security and to some extent neighbours and relatives. (Asian Bangladeshi woman)

> I would get, and give, support in a situation whereby where it didn't necessarily interfere with somebody's life, but if you're talking total incapacity, I wouldn't expect friends to do it and I wouldn't do it for friends. I'd expect the state to do it. (White British/Irish man)

Participants with direct experience of this nexus suggested that pragmatism was more important than intellectual or emotional adherence to an ideal:

> Actually, I think your family should support you but . . . they've got their own share of things to do and I think the state or council or whatever it is should provide . . . I cannot pinpoint [one single responsibility]. The fact is I think it's nice to be independent because I have seen in my life, you know, [children's attitudes] one day [older people] are good, the next day, they are burden. (Asian Indian woman)

Only a minority favoured models in which families took total responsibility for supporting older members and, in most cases, these were people who had little direct experience of either giving or receiving care.

People from minority ethnic groups are generally less likely to either be aware of, or to be offered, health and social care services than their white counterparts (Ahmad and Atkin 1996; Butt and Mirza 1996). Although almost two-thirds of participants had a long-standing illness or disability that affected their everyday lives, only 42 per cent were currently using one or more of the following health and social care services: home care, day care, meals, lunch clubs, community nurses, community psychiatric nurses, social workers, occupational therapy, physiotherapy, chiropody, and welfare rights and benefits. However, unlike the two other studies reported in this chapter, participants were less concerned that using services would compromise their independence or privacy, it was simply that they had rarely been given an opportunity to consider using them in the first place.

141

Earlier research has examined the extent to which older people manage their identity as consumers of health and social care services through the purchase of care privately (Baldock and Ungerson 1994; Wilson 1994; Ungerson 1999). Strikingly, just 16 participants had arranged and paid for help themselves. Of these, only two used someone to provide personal care. Eight of them were white, suggesting that if the policy of providing additional flexibility through direct payments (Department of Health 2003) is to be successful, attention must be paid to ensuring that there are no barriers that prevent people from minority ethnic groups from choosing this option.

Meaning and purpose in life

Almost a third of participants described relationships with their family as something that made their life good and gave it meaning. Another tenth mentioned aspects relating to their wider social network. For some people, family support helped them to cope with difficulties such as ill health:

> If the family is good . . . you don't face all these problems too much . . . You can get depressed, or you can get any problem, if you haven't got any family support. If everybody had family support, there would be no problems . . . Maybe I'm the lucky one! (Asian Indian man)

For others, being in good health or having an adequate income could not compensate for its absence:

> My son . . . has informed me I've got no right to feel miserable because I live in a comfortable home and I've got sufficient income . . . but it's not just having money and having a warm [house] and enough to eat. That isn't what makes life good. (White British woman)

Some participants did not see strong demarcations between their own identity and those of their family. This was especially true of some Asian women with lives centred on the home. This was the interview topic that interested them most and they spoke with a fluency and enthusiasm less evident in their answers elsewhere: 'I'm happy that I don't have any sadness and my daughters are well. They don't have any problems. All three are healthy and happy, so I'm happy' (Asian Indian woman).

Ageing and identity

Biggs (1997, 2004) has identified growing interest in the relationship between ageing and identity in later life exemplified in the viewpoint that clearly defined stages of the lifecourse are becoming blurred and being replaced by multiple consumerist identities (Featherstone and Hepworth 1993; Gilleard and Higgs 2000). However, Biggs also points out that much of this discussion has been theoretically driven and that we need a better understanding of the layering of ageing identities and the intersection of age, gender, ethnicity and class.

Almost half the participants associated growing older with illness or disability. Others mentioned other negative experiences such as the loss of independence or isolation. However, the extent to which they felt this affected their QoL varied considerably. In particular, many participants had developed different strategies to cope with physical changes:

> You know I really love dancing . . . I used to do Bhangra . . . I'm the first one to go on the dance floor but when I see these two things [pointing to knees] . . . I say, 'Oh if I'm going to go on there, what will happen? I may fall now with my pain' . . . I love [listening to] music all day . . . If I'm upset I put the music on for a minute and I'll forget my pain. (Asian Indian woman)

Other approaches included maintaining an internal sense of achievement or spiritual comfort. There were also those who saw ageing as bringing advantages as well as disadvantages:

> You move on. You know, you don't stay stagnant and one has got to be grateful that you reached a certain age. You go through a process. You've made mistakes and you are able to correct it and pass on the correction to the younger generation. That is old age. (Mixed White and Black Caribbean man)

Overall, participants from minority ethnic groups expressed more positive attitudes towards ageing than their white counterparts. While some viewpoints, such as the layering of identity or the experience of ageism upon the sense of self, are similar to examples found in the existing literature (which is largely based upon the experiences of white people), they were more inclined to see ageing as a normal part of life, rather than a pathological process:

> I haven't thought about that, you know, cos getting old is part of life so I don't take much notice of it. (Black African woman)

> A person ages from youth . . . [when you are young] they say, 'You are young, oh, don't you look good' but as you age [they say] 'Oh, she's gone old, she's finished.' (Laughs) It's the truth, isn't it? [Ageing] is inevitable but they [the young] don't think that they will grow old too. (Asian Indian woman)

The role of past experience

The study suggested that, across all ethnic groups, social support made an important contribution to QoL and gave it a sense of meaning and purpose.

Participants did not see the advent of illness or disability as automatically pre-cluding them from providing as well as receiving support. The overwhelming majority were strongly committed to the notion of state responsibility for care in old age and, contrary to many stereotyped perceptions, participants from minority ethnic groups rarely saw help from health and social care services as automatically inferior to family care; the real barrier was that it was rare for this help to have been offered.

It also raised questions about the impact of previous life experiences. In particular, there was a sense of inevitability about ageing and acceptance that it was likely to involve changes, both positive and negative, that enabled people from minority ethnic groups to approach their own ageing with some degree of equanimity. For this generation, the experience of migration has already involved them in making major adaptations to their life and they have possibly acquired a sense of adaptability that has stood them in good stead, as they have grown older. Equally, their experiences may have encouraged them to have lower expectations (Tsang et al. 2004). Some participants had undergone very difficult life events and they saw their old age as qualitatively better than earlier parts of their lives. However, the question remains as to whether these differences will remain or whether there will be greater convergence between the views of participants from different ethnic groups in the future.

Conclusion: social support and identity

The connections between social support and sense of self in older people operate in a variety of ways. Receiving and providing social support can reinforce identity through the possibilities that this offers for material and symbolic exchange. Thus, for some people, supporting or being supported by a partner was (despite the tensions it could create) a 'natural' part of a long-standing affective relationship and reflected on as affirming the validity of the relationship and self as a partner in that relationship. Giving and receiving support could also be seen to transform one's sense of self, as an individual's perceived role within a relationship appeared to have been inverted, with those used to being the giver of support being transformed into receivers, and vice versa. Inability to interact socially because of lack of mobility affected the sense of self for some people who described themselves as having been transformed from one type of person to another, for example, from a gregarious person into an isolated individual. In some cases, using formal support services was felt to challenge individuals' identity by reinforcing the unwelcome sense that they had been transformed from independent adults able to exercise their own choices into a person dependent on others. Some were able to accommodate this transformation within a framework of ageing seen inevitably to entail decline. Others did not cite a particular view of what ageing means and saw the rejection of services as a way of reasserting themselves as adults, able to make choices for themselves, even in apparently minor ways such as deciding what to eat, and what time to dress for bed.

Old age, particularly when accompanied by a loss of independence is, indeed, a period when people engage in identity work in order to sustain and develop their conceptions of self and maintain self-esteem. Becoming more dependent can have a marked downward effect on self-esteem. The best immediate protections against this are forms of inner emotional strength such as spirituality or belief in one's capacity to overcome new limitations. People do adjust to constraints and dependencies. Marked improvements in self-esteem often occur following outside interventions. Most people's sense of well-being and self-esteem will rise in the months after the shock of new dependency. However, the older people in our samples rarely saw interventions by professional providers of services as a potential source of improvement. We found evidence that increased contact with others rather than specific forms of help is most likely to improve self-esteem. Overall the findings suggest that there are limits to the degree to which older people's conceptions of their circumstances and needs can be reconciled with those of potential service providers. The gaps between models that inform medical and social care practitioners in their work with older people and the lay conceptions of the older people themselves are real. However, they may also be necessary and inevitable. The notion of a reconciliation between the perspectives of producers and users of care services is superficially attractive, however, it is unclear what would be gained. Neither 'side' is wrong in their perceptions and in our samples we could see examples where the tension between them had been productive. Where appropriate, formal service providers should intervene early to increase an older person's contact with others. There may be resistance from the older person, but this will be because she or he has other work to do: maintaining and strengthening an identity and values built up across almost a whole lifetime.

10

Elderly bereaved spouses
Issues of belief, well-being and support

Peter Speck, Kate M. Bennett, Peter G. Coleman,
Marie Mills, Fionnuala McKiernan, Philip T. Smith and
Georgina M. Hughes

Introduction

The death of someone with whom you have spent a lifetime will lead to a variety of reactions and feelings within the person 'left behind'. Over the years, the way in which people seek to re-build their life following the death of a spouse or partner has been the focus of much research. The models that have been developed have been replaced or significantly re-shaped over the years. The current focus on the need to find meaning within the event for the ongoing life of the survivor, and the emphasis on gender are important developments which have influenced the two studies into the experience of older bereaved spouses we describe in this chapter.

Models and theories

It is important to clarify some of the terms we shall use within this chapter. Bereavement is the objective situation or state of having experienced the death of someone significant in one's life. Grief is the emotional response and feelings that are expressed, following that loss, and is therefore highly individualized. The term 'mourning' relates to the actions and way in which grief is expressed. This is often shaped by the practices, culture or beliefs of the group to which the person belongs. Within modern society there is great emphasis on the individual and, as Walter (1999) indicates, individual diversity is paramount so that, within broad constraints, each of us develops our own way of 'doing' bereavement and grief. This matches well the experience of many bereavement workers who find that most of their clients have not read the theory, do not follow a prescribed path, but get on with doing their own thing. Many healthcare professionals have had to 'unlearn' much that they were taught years ago as current research has challenged existing practices. The main models that were developed ranged through the 'phase' model, the 'medical' model, the 'grief work' model, the 'biographical' and the 'dual-process' model. Each of these had their merits as well as limitations.

In the *phase model* it is envisaged that the bereaved person moves over time through a series of phases, the number and description of which vary for different authors. Thus, Elizabeth Kubler-Ross (1990) talks of five stages, Bowlby (1981) and Parkes (1996) of four and others of eight. Such phases are to be seen as a classification of the reactions and not prescriptive for grief. Unfortunately, people have tended to take Kubler-Ross's stages as sequential and steer people through them in the 'right' order. While grief is seen as a process in this model, in reality, people will move back and forth until they achieve some form of resolution.

The *medical model* sees all grief as pathological, or at the very least an illness, which is painful and requires appropriate treatment. Here the process is 'pathologized' and may be treated as a 'reactive' depression requiring medication. In some ways the concept of 'compassionate' leave seems to mirror this model. The few days allowed are inadequate to make funeral arrangements, let alone adjust to what has happened. In order to make proper arrangements for and attend a funeral (in the UK), extra time off work is required. This is usually provided for, via the family doctor, by being signed off sick – with depression.

The *grief work model* is based on Freud's work on mourning and melancholia, where it is acknowledged that we need time to test reality without the deceased being around. We should not avoid doing this psychological work in the immediate aftermath, as well as later, for the sake of our future mental health. In many ways, Worden (2003) develops this in his 'tasks of mourning' which, in contrast to a more passive engagement with phases, encourages the bereaved to actively engage with four tasks.

Walter's *biographical model* (1996) develops the idea that people benefit from talking to others about the deceased person and their life. This provides a way of the bereaved 'keeping hold' of the dead so that their memory is a continuous presence. This model encourages living with the past in order to gain strength to face the future.

Stroebe and colleagues (1993) advocate, on the basis of their research, a *dual-process model* whereby the bereaved oscillate over time between confronting and avoiding reality. Sometimes they will be very engaged in tasks and seemingly not in touch with feelings, and at other times they will be consumed by the pain of grief.

All these models have a theoretical basis which shapes them and explains the underlying reasons for the observed behaviours to assist others in making appropriate and helpful interventions. These different theories complement each other as each contributes to our understanding of the similarities and differences between individual and group responses to bereavement. In particular, they are supported by research evidence and have not been formed from anecdotal sources. However, they have not been without challenge, especially in relation to the idea of a linear progression through stages or phases and the necessity of grief work (Wortman and Silver 1989). In a critique, Bennett and Bennett (2000–2001) argue that bereaved spouses themselves are uncomfortable with these approaches. First, these theories may, often unintentionally, suggest that grief is a pathological experience, rather than one which is a normal experience, arising from the common experience of spousal bereavement in later life. Second, that stage theories suggest, again often unintentionally, that there is a specific way and process which are beneficial. Widows believe that this is unhelpful and prescriptive. These authors suggest that there are enormous individual differences in the ways in which people grieve and deal with their bereavement.

Age and gender, as factors influencing bereavement outcome, have also been the subject of debate. Martin and Doka (1998) suggest that many of the gender differences in approach to grief may be more to do with socialization than intrinsic genetic differences. Doka (1989) also introduced the idea of 'grieving rules' which operate as a subset of the 'feeling' rules which exist in each society (Hochschild 1979). If a person grieves outside of these rules, their grief may be disenfranchised since the rules determine what losses can be grieved for and how the individual may express that grief. The faith community can be very influential in respect of this. Men are seen as more likely to be at the instrumental end of the spectrum, while women are more likely to show an intuitive style. The grieving rules vary according to ethnicity, gender, age and class, with the very old being allowed more latitude for expression.

Religion can be important in providing a framework for the mourner to understand and express their grief. This fact has been recognized by many including Gorer (1965) and Hinton (1967) who felt that the decline in accepted ritual, religious guidance and support in bereavement contributed to maladaptive behaviour later. The need to understand the event and make sense of what has happened is a developing one in bereavement research which is often expressed as the search for meaning (Fry 1998). Traumatic events have the power to disrupt our personal interpretations of reality and the belief system we hold, so that we may need to restructure that belief in order to create new meaning (Braun and Berg 1994). Research into the role of religious and spiritual belief and bereavement has been limited by the tendency to look at religious behaviour and practice as the measure of spiritual belief. Against a backcloth of many who no longer give religious expression to their beliefs, this is no longer appropriate. Stroebe and Stroebe (1987) incorporated a religiosity scale into their bereavement study to assess the impact of religious beliefs and habits on coping with loss. Although nearly half of their sample were sufficiently religious to believe in an after-life, these beliefs did not seem to help them cope with their loss experience (see also Lund et al. 1993).

In the first of the studies we describe in this chapter we have drawn on recent work by King et al. (2001), who have developed a measure for the strength of spiritual belief that allows us to look for correlations with a variety of bereavement outcomes. By differentiating between religion and spirituality, while recognizing their inter-relatedness, we believe that the broader spiritual belief might influence the outcome in bereavement.

The Southampton study

The Southampton study was a prospective case study of older people bereaved in the previous 12–15 months. The study was an exploratory one and we did not attempt to provide representative data, but rich descriptions of the issues that arise relating to belief and support for belief following bereavement. We therefore chose to use a case study methodology, following up cases over a one-year period, interviewing three times, beginning after the first anniversary of the death, then six months later, and finally after the second anniversary: For each case we investigated evidence on the person's adjustment to bereavement, the role of belief systems in that adjustment, and support for those belief systems. In addition, we considered each individual's need for counselling and support, including pastoral care.

Our cases were drawn from GPs' and funeral directors' lists in three cities/towns in the South of England. Acceptances were low (34 per cent), but comparable to other studies on bereavement, and it proved particularly difficult to recruit men to the study. Over a period of four months we recruited 28 people to the study (22 women + 6 men), and have been successful in interviewing three times, over the one-year study period, all but two of these people.

The age range of our sample was from 61 to 89 years, with a mean age of 74 years. The sample varied considerably in physical health, including a significant number with physical and/or mental health problems. All our sample came from a Christian background. The measures used included the Royal Free Interview – strength of belief scale (King et al. 2001). To assess perception of meaning we used the Life-Attitude Profile (Reker 1996) which contains no religiously worded items and is therefore useful in investigating the meaning-enhancing qualities of spiritual and non-spiritual beliefs. We also employed a 45-item Bereavement Experience Index (Carr and McKiernan) recently developed by another member of Southampton team, plus the well-established Short Form 36 health survey (SF36), the Geriatric Depression Scale (GDS), and the Southampton Self-Esteem and Sources of Self-Esteem Scale. Particular attention was paid to the dialogues of questioning and answering in which the person engaged, both in terms of internal thought processes (the dialogical self – Hermans et al. (1992)) and external conversation with significant others, relating to the deceased person, his or her meaning for the person's own life, and the continuing purpose and significance of living.

Results

The sample showed an even distribution across the three categories of strength of spiritual belief that we employed. This referred to belief in an external power operative in their personal lives and in the world in general. Nine (32 per cent) indicated low or weak spiritual belief, 11 (39 per cent) moderate levels of belief, and eight (29 per cent) strong belief. All those of strong belief attended church, prayed and believed in life after death. None of those of weak or no belief attended church, prayed or believed in life after death. By contrast, all of the moderate group prayed, but only a minority of them attended church or believed in life after death. All nine people in the strong belief group, and nine of the 11 in the moderate group described their beliefs as religious, the remaining two described themselves as spiritual but not religious.

The term 'spiritual' appeared to make some of the sample uncomfortable, perhaps because of the associations with spiritualism in the minds of this generation of older people. 'Religion' was defined as the practice of a particular faith. Although most of the sample has been brought up with a religious faith – virtually all of the sample, for example, had attended Sunday School – large numbers had doubts or misunderstandings about central tenets of the Christian faith, such as the doctrine of the Trinity, the divine and human nature of Christ, and the power of God over evil. Many were troubled by the problem of a good God who could allow suffering. Yet very few outside of the church attenders were in contact with ministers or spoke about issues of spiritual belief with church members.

Belief and adjustment to bereavement

A remarkably strong association was found between strength of belief and adjustment to bereavement. For this analysis we averaged scores on the measure of strength of spiritual beliefs for the two occasions and rank ordered them. All those of strong belief displayed scores above the norm for their age group on both personal meaning and existential transcendence. None displayed above criterion depression scores or gave significant indications of mental health problems.

Depressive symptoms were concentrated among those of moderate to weak belief. A significant number of this group also indicated below the norm scores on both personal meaning and existential transcendence. However, it is note-worthy that some people of moderate, weak and no spiritual belief scored high on these scales too, which demonstrates the independence of the measures of personal meaning and spiritual belief.

This is the pattern of results we expected. It accords with previous studies, for example, which show that death anxiety is concentrated among those of moderate levels of belief, and justifies our particular interest in the moderate believers. Of the 11 people identified as moderate believers, eight indicated low levels of personal meaning and all but one of these displayed depressive symp-toms during the second year after bereavement. All provide evidence on the unsatisfactory nature of their beliefs and its association with low perceived meaning in their lives. For example, one 65-year-old widow attends her local parish church in the hope of cultivating belief and envies believers their faith. She hopes someone is listening to her prayers, but is more inclined to believe in the operation of a 'cold fate'. As she grows older, she feels she believes less and less, and in this thinks that she is contrary to the norm. She is disillusioned by human nature, and states that she is not at peace with her beliefs. Another participant, a widower who is also 65 years old, says that he likes to sit quietly in church but outside service times, having an antipathy towards church authority. He prays regularly, 'feeling he owes someone something', and finds it helpful, especially following his bereavement. Although religion means more to him now that he is older – especially the moral teaching contained in the Bible – he cannot see God as a person or Jesus as God. He would like to understand more.

Some had encountered difficulties sustaining their beliefs following the loss of spouse. A widow of 63 years has suffered a double bereavement of mother and husband, the latter after 17 years caring for him with chronic illness. She became depressed and admits her faith was initially shaken by these events. She thought that she would get more comfort from her faith, yet at the same time she considers that she could not have coped without it. She has continued to attend her local parish church throughout, and thinks well of it. Her depression has now diminished, and she has a high sense of personal meaning, although her strength of spiritual belief remains moderate. She has questions about God and in particular cannot understand how He allows cruelty. Still she believes that God is 'stronger than the world's wickedness'.

Most of our participants of moderate or low belief had little or no contact with their local churches. As noted already, many had difficulty articulating both their beliefs and doubts, but appreciated the opportunity to be encouraged to do so. It is significant that most of the sample – including therefore also those of weak or no belief – would have appreciated some pastoral interest expressed in them by their local church following bereavement. A form of contact, which all would have accepted, would have been a card with a contact telephone number put through their letter-box.

Examination of these case studies of moderate believers provides suggestive evidence on the importance of doubts about belief to low personal meaning in the current generation of older people. Moreover, lack of integration into the religious structures appears related to depressed responses following bereavement. As they have become older and more housebound, several complained of being 'neglected' by the Church. Isolation from the religion of origin is likely to be a common experience and one which some at least regret.

Yet there is still hesitancy on the part of health and welfare agencies to engage with the Churches. Religion and spirituality remain something of a taboo subject and one which professionals find difficult to approach in a sensitive and appropriate manner. Practice, within care settings, is often limited to ticking a faith or denomination box, without further enquiries into the implications for practical help and counselling. Re-engaging with older people is not an easy task for Churches either. As our interviews also illustrate, some people have concerns about the authority exerted by the clergy that they have experienced in the past. There is also no uniform acceptance of the character of religious service or liturgy. Yet, compared with young people, older people have at least had a religious background – most have attended Sunday School – which provides a starting point for contact and further exploration. Profound questions concerning the nature of belief and the meaning of life arise as people age, yet most commonly questioning appears to be experienced in isolation rather than in dialogue with another person.

The study demonstrates that, although not without difficulties, it is possible to engage older people in a discussion of their spiritual beliefs, especially if the interview is rooted in their accounts of daily experience. Our data provide a striking demonstration of the association between beliefs and experience of well-being. There are important issues here for religious organizations and we are attempting to elucidate some of them in further research.

We are continuing to investigate older people's views of belief and the role of religious organizations and broadening the scope of our work to include not only different Christian denominations but the major faith communities living in Britain today, and forms of meaning-giving fellowship and spiritual belief that exist outside of the major religious traditions.

The Liverpool study

The Liverpool study aimed to investigate the influence of gender and widowhood on well-being and lifestyle in later life. We interviewed 46 widowed men and 46 women aged between 55 and 95 years (mean = 74) living in the North-West of England. They had been widowed between three months to 60 years (mean 9.5 years). In order to recruit, the aims of the Older Widow(er)s Project were communicated to a diverse range of formal and informal groups of older people. Recruitment issues are discussed in more detail later in this chapter. The interviews were conducted by one of three interviewers and were tape-recorded, took place at the respondents' homes, at a day centre or at the University of Liverpool and lasted between one and two hours.

The interviews were semi-structured and were designed to elicit information on lifestyle and affect, by asking what the participants did and how they felt at specific times. Respondents were first asked factual information concerning age, length of marriage, widowhood and family relations. Second, participants were essentially asked two questions (with supplementary questions) about their widowhood; what did you do?; and how did you feel? These two questions were asked repeatedly following the chronology of events: married life prior to widowhood; the time around the death of the spouse; one year post-bereavement (for those who had been widowed for longer); and the present time.

Results

The data presented here examine issues which surround personal meaning, church attendance and spiritual beliefs. The study did not set out to directly discuss these issues with participants, nevertheless these were issues which arose in the interviews.

In previous work by Bennett on widowed people in the East Midlands, religion and church attendance were not a significant factor in interviews (Bennett and Bennett 2000–2001). The interviews in Liverpool were in marked contrast. As Peter Speck explained to a GO project meeting with the Liverpool group, Liverpool is a religious city. Some 42 per cent of the participants attended church, and several more attended luncheon clubs or other social clubs organized by churches such as the Salvation Army, Church of England and Non-Conformist churches; 23 per cent discussed issues of faith, and three of faith change.

A number of themes emerged. First, there were participants whose faith remained steady as did their church attendance, and a subset who found their faith very supportive following their bereavement. Second, there were those whose allegiance changed as a consequence of their bereavement. Finally, there were those without religious belief who discussed issues of personal meaning in relationship to their bereavement.

A number of participants found that their faith remained steady throughout the events associated with bereavement. These were participants who were regular and active church members. Man 28 said, 'I go to church Sunday morning – yes, I go to communion.' Both men and women attended church, and many were involved in more church activities. For example, Man 23 said, 'We always went to church on Sunday . . . Still go regularly to church . . . We was quite involved in the Church.' These quotes also show the range of denominations that people belong to:

I mean, I'm at the [Salvation] Army at least three times a week. (Man 8)

Because we were always in church on Sundays. (Woman 29)

I'm a Catholic and I go to church. Belong to the Mothers Union. (Woman 31)

Some of these participants also described how their faith assisted them during their bereavement:

It's just that I believe there is a god and he listens to you even in times of distress. (Man 23)

He's in the communion of Saints . . . and I don't think that means halos. No. It just means kind of fellowship of the church. (Woman 6)

I went every morning and every evening, like, I say prayers . . . you have a period of mourning for your wife of a month. (Man 4)

This last quote is from one of two Jewish participants. It is clear that for these participants above that their faith and church involvement were important to them in providing some meaning or support when confronting the painful realization that their partner had died.

Second, there were a small number of participants whose faith changed as a consequence of bereavement, either in terms of their allegiance to a particular denomination or who began to doubt their beliefs. Returning to Man 21, he had been a church attendee as a young man, but had not attended regularly for some time. He spoke about an encounter with the Vicar: 'As a result of chatting with him I went back to church . . . It's, you know amazing.' One woman explicitly discussed her change in denominational allegiance, and this was also an issue for other participants, though less explicit: 'I still go to church but, um, then the more I go to the Army, the more I wanted to go and do more as well. Yes. So, finally, I enrolled' (Woman 1).

There are interesting aspects to Woman 1. First, the move appears to always be towards involvement in the Salvation Army through attendance at social organizations which were either run by or accommodated by the Salvation Army. Second, it is also the case that this change in faith and allegiance does not occur as single event. Attendance at one church does not preclude attendance at another.

There was also one explicit discussion of the loss of faith and the attempts to maintain that faith. Woman 46 said, 'Yes, I tried for 12 months, I really tried and I got no comfort whatsoever.'

Finally, there were also people who, while having no religious or spiritual beliefs, experienced personal growth and changes, what we would call augmentation of identity. For the most part, these participants were women rather than men. For example, Woman 32 identifies the change from being one of two to being one: 'That was when I started to become me instead of us' (Woman 32). Other women talked about personal development and the acquisition of confidence: 'I think you get a bit more confident when you are on your own, cos you know you've got things to do' (Woman 45). In addition, women also point to personal growth in the sense of the ability to choose what things to do and when to do them: 'Now life's completely changed because I just do things when I want to do them' (Woman 18).

The Liverpool study has shown that widowed people draw on spiritual and secular resources in order to provide meaning to their lives and to ensure that something positive emerges from what is otherwise a devastating and apparently pointless event, the death of one's spouse. People employ both external and internal mechanisms in order to achieve this, whether they are spiritual and personal beliefs, or church attendance and new secular activities.

Some practical considerations

Reflections on the process of obtaining approval from the research ethics committee

Obtaining ethical approval from the research ethics committee (REC) is not always a straightforward process, however well the protocol has been prepared. Recent studies within palliative care (Stevens et al. 2004) have shown that RECs tend to be over-protective of potential participants for studies into end-of-life care, elderly care and bereavement. There can also be a suspicion that psychological studies carry a high risk of distress for participants. There would seem to be a need to develop the understanding of committee members concerning qualitative methodology and the acceptability of such studies to participants. In part, this can be addressed by involving users of services in the study design and by undertaking a small pilot with an exit audit, the results of which can accompany the main application for approval. As indicated above, the appropriateness of the researchers' background training and experience can feature highly in the REC scrutiny of proposals.

The Southampton study, plus other recent work, indicates that religious needs are not fully met in later life. Coleman et al. (2004), Howse (1999), and Speck (in press) argue that older people are quite capable of discussing beliefs and religious/spiritual needs with an experienced and sympathetic interviewer. This places demands on the researcher/interviewer who is required to have the necessary understanding and skills to undertake such work. These skills include knowledge of the ageing process, and an understanding of a variety of religious beliefs and practices suited to the area under investigation.

It is also suggested that the interviewer should have received specific training when the topic under investigation is highly sensitive in nature (Coleman et al.

2002; Mills 2002). Most qualitative studies of beliefs in later life find that beliefs tend to be discussed against their effectiveness as coping measures in times of crisis. Some older people find this difficult and will want to be reassured that their story or narrative will be sympathetically heard, even if the recruitment and investigation are conducted at a distance, for example, by postal questionnaire or telephone interview.

The personal narrative is inextricably interlinked with life and meaning (Sarbin 1986). We believe that disclosing one's beliefs or moral narrative to self, or to an understanding other, encourages the development of meaning and understanding (Vitz 1990) and is often therapeutic in itself.

Selection issues

Studies of widowhood, especially those using interviews, present a number of methodological challenges concerning selection. First, this type of work is only possible, and indeed ethical, with volunteers. Second, there is a danger that those who volunteer are not representative of the widowed population as a whole. For instance, participants who volunteer for interview studies may be those who are more articulate or who may have a particular agenda of their own regarding widowhood. Third, the sample size for qualitative interview studies is usually smaller than for quantitative work, and, as a consequence, the claims made by such studies are different. Finally, widowed people do not represent a homogeneous social group. In both studies we considered these issues carefully and addressed them as far as is possible. Addressing the first two issues together, we engaged in extensive out-reach work to ensure that we did not recruit only those widowed people who always participate. Indeed, virtually all of our participants had not taken part in research before, many were recruited by word of mouth, or encouraged to participate by friends or support networks. It is clear from our transcripts that many of our participants were not highly articulate or well educated. Participants came from a wide range of social and economic backgrounds, representing the diversity of our respective areas. Indeed, for the Liverpool study we compared our sample with national norms and found no significant differences. In Liverpool we were able to recruit equal numbers of men and women, despite the general difficulties found by other researchers to do so. Unfortunately our samples did not reflect ethnic diversity, although we did try. The heterogeneity of the samples is, we believe, a strength. The sample reflected all socioeconomic statuses and was also diverse with respect to age and length of time widowed.

Gender issues

Another issue which warrants some discussion is the issue of the charac-teristics of interviewer and interviewee. The interviewee–interviewer charac-teristics which may be important include gender, ethnicity, age, class, marital status, and, in the context of the issues discussed earlier, religious outlook. We will discuss two of these briefly: gender and age. In both studies the major-ity of the interviews were conducted by women. In the Southampton study the majority of participants were women, but in Liverpool there were equal numbers of women and men. In another study of men living alone, Arber, Davidson et al. (2003) used both male and female interviewers and found that some issues were discussed more openly with men while others were discussed more openly with women. We did not get a sense from our interviews that male participants were holding back, even when discussing such issues as repartnering or intimacy. Age is also an issue which could be influential. In both studies the majority of the interviews were conducted by mature women. In the Liverpool study about 10 per cent were conducted by a woman in her late thirties. There did not appear to be a difference in the quality of the interviews between these two ages. However, these issues are worthy of more research.

Interviewer considerations

There are two issues which are important in what might be considered 'health and safety': physical safety and maintaining the psychological well-being of interviewers. Taking the first issue, many of our respondents chose to be inter-viewed in their own homes. Interviewers are invited into people's homes and one works on the basis of trust, that is, that no harm will come to the inter-viewer. On occasions, however, an interviewer might feel uncomfortable if, for example, personal space is invaded or an interviewee behaves inappropriately or is aggressive. Fortunately these situations have been extremely rare. It is important though to ensure that there are procedures in place to protect the interviewer. For example, someone else should always know where an inter-view is taking place, a mobile phone can be left on, and the interviewer should make contact with another member of the team when the interview finishes. With respect to the psychological well-being of the interviewer, it needs to be remembered that interviewing people about bereavement is psychologically challenging and draining. As in clinical practice, it is important that regular debriefing takes place. In addition, it is better that no more than two interviews take place a day and no more than five a week. If the interviewer has experienced their own loss, then someone else should do the interviews.

Conclusion

There are two conclusions which we would like to draw. The first concerns theoretical developments which these two studies have facilitated. The second concerns the key practical issue of conducting research in an environment which is safe for both participant and researcher.

Both studies have demonstrated that there is a fundamental need for some bereaved people to tell their stories. Bennett and Vidal-Hall (2000) found that widowed participants talked at great length about their experience of bereavement and that it appeared to serve many functions including remembrance, respect for their dead husbands, and establishing self-identity. The studies presented in this chapter show that an additional function of narrative is the development of identity. Our participants demonstrated through their discussions of spirituality and personal growth the ways in which their identities were shifting as a consequence of their bereavement experiences. Bennett et al. (submitted) have suggested that widowed people do not adopt a new identity, rather that their identity is augmented to encompass that of wife/husband with that of widow/widower. In the data presented here that augmentation is influenced by both internal and external resources which are based on issues of spiritual belief and personal self-worth. Internal resources include faith, spirituality and personal ideals and beliefs. External resources include church attendance, support from religious leaders and congregations, and support from family and social networks. People do not fall necessarily into either a category of spiritual or secular. Rather it appears that they are on a continuum and draw from whatever resource they need as their psychological and indeed practical needs require it.

In terms of the practical issues, our key observation concerns that of the safety of the research encounter. We mean safety in the broadest sense. Participants need to feel safe, their experience needs to be treated with confidentiality and respect. It is important that they are not deserted by researchers when they are feeling emotionally vulnerable. Interview encounters should not be left on an emotionally raw note. It is also the case that researchers should also work in a safe environment. They should not be put in situations where they are at physical risk. In addition, there should be opportunities for debriefing, not only for those conducting interviews but also for those transcribing or coding interviews and indeed for those writing up results – these people are not always the same.

The experience of conducting research into bereavement has been a very rewarding one. As researchers we have learned a great deal not only about the ways to conduct such sensitive research but more importantly we have gained greater knowledge about the lives of older bereaved people that have enabled us to develop theoretical insights into the psychological and spiritual experiences associated with bereavement in later life.

11

Conclusion

From research to action

Alan Walker

This book and its companions in the GO series contain a wealth of empirical information about the quality of life (QoL) of older people and the host of factors that contribute to it. Nonetheless, as noted in Chapter 1, one volume cannot possibly contain all of the data and analyses produced by such a massive undertaking. The largest social science research programme on ageing ever mounted in the UK has, as the previous chapters demonstrate, told us a great deal about the quality of later life. The question that hangs in the air from the introduction to the first volume in this series (Walker 2004) is, will this huge body of evidence be translated into real QoL improvements for older people? Whether it will or not is beyond the control of those involved in the GO Programme but, perhaps, not beyond their influence, which is why the Programme made such extraordinary efforts to deliver its findings to the policy and practice communities. Nonetheless the question remains and is of concern to all researchers working in the ageing field and not only those responsible for the GO projects. Needless to say, it is of greatest personal interest to older people themselves who bear the cost if, to paraphrase the World Health Organization (WHO), their extra years are not filled with quality life. Many policy-makers, practitioners and organizations representing older people are also keenly interested in trying to improve the quality of later life. Therefore, this volume will conclude with some reflections on the link between research and policy and practice. First, it will look at why population ageing has moved up the policy agenda in the last decade and, with it, funding for research on this topic.

The rising importance of ageing as a policy issue

The first factor in explaining the emergence of population ageing as a major policy issue in all developed countries is demography itself. Ageing is a global phenomenon and Europe has aged in advance of most other regions of the world. The combination of declining birth rates and declining death rates means that there are fewer young people and more older ones. In the language of demography, the population pyramid is bulging and fast becoming cone shaped. This is unprecedented in human history and presents unique challenges to all aspects of society, from the labour market to family life, from the health service to political parties and the institutions of democratic participation, in short, to every aspect of social, economic and political life. For example the trebling of the numbers of people aged 80 and over in the EU, in the next 25 years, is an outstanding example of social and economic progress but it raises profound questions about both caring relationships within families and the social contract between the generations on which the EU's pensions, health and social care systems are based (Walker 1997a, 2005a).

Demographic pressures alone are not sufficient to explain the increased policy profile of ageing nor the growth in welfare state spending on older people. Looking at the post-war growth of spending on older people in all advanced industrial societies, demography accounts for only one-third of the rise with the vast bulk of the increase being due to policy changes (OECD 1988). In the UK, until the late 1970s, governments of both major political parties were willing to fund increases in pensions and health services for older people, not in response to demographic change but in order to improve QoL and to try to overcome the poverty and deprivation that a large proportion of older people were experiencing. The same is true in other EU countries and the growth of public spending on older people was even greater in other comparable countries than in the UK (Walker and Maltby 1997).

However, the relatively privileged position that older people occupied in the eyes of policy-makers in the previous post-war decades began to be reversed in the 1980s with the UK leading the way. Not only were big cuts made in public pensions but, also, these changes were accompanied by negative political rhetoric about the 'burden' of ageing and the economic costs of pensions (Walker 1990). It is very difficult to over-estimate the importance of those policy changes in the 1980s. It is also important to emphasize how far the UK was out of step with the rest of the EU in this policy direction. Comparatively speaking, it was much closer to Japan and the USA, both of which carried out major pension reforms in the 1980s (Myles and Quadagno 1993). Most of the other EU countries began to implement their own reform programmes in the 1990s but, so far, none of them have been as extreme, in terms of pension reductions, as in the UK.

The 1990s brought new policy concerns. First of all, the so-called 'demographic timebomb' of falling numbers of young labour market entrants. Of course, this was no more than the work-force reflecting the general ageing of the population but it led to a flurry of public statements. By 2015 the proportion of the total EU workforce aged 50 and over will rise from one-fifth to over one-quarter. The implications of this ageing of the work-force have been addressed so far by very few employers but their numbers are increasing slowly (Walker and Taylor 1998). Gradually EU governments are realizing the importance of work-force ageing (Walker 1997b). In fact, the EU itself has played an important role in pushing this item up the policy agenda. For example, the European Councils in 1998 and 1999 emphasized the need to sustain employment among older workers and, in 2000, the Employment Guidelines which are the key method of coordinating the policies of the Member States in this field, contained the first explicit references for the employment of older workers. A key development in this EU action was the resolution on older workers introduced by the French Presidency in 1995. Active ageing has emerged as a major policy priority within the EU but is also being promoted by other big players on the global scene, such as the Organization for Economic Cooperation and Development (OECD) and the G8. Activity in this context means mainly economic activity but the other policy concerns have helped to broaden the meaning of active ageing (WHO 2001a, 2001b; Walker 2002).

The second major policy issue to emerge in the 1990s was that of social care. The fastest growing segment of the older population is those over 80 and, between 2000 and 2005, an 18 per cent increase in this age group was projected for the EU as a whole. The realization that population ageing meant the likelihood of increasing demands for social care has resulted in policy action in most EU countries, notably the introduction of long-term care insurance in Germany. In the UK the need for urgency on this front was reinforced by the cost of the perverse incentive introduced by the Conservative Government in the mid-1980s for older people to enter residential homes rather than staying put, and the need for some of them to sell their family homes in order to receive social security subsidies. Also the campaigns by groups representing older people and carers helped to raise the profile of this issue as well as achieving important social advances such as the Carers Act (1996). The first Royal

Commission for a decade was appointed to look into this issue (The Royal Commission on Long-Term Care 1999) and led to some important changes although not the most important one, the provision of free personal care, as recommended by the Commission. This reform was implemented in Scotland.

A by-product of this policy focus on social care was the revival of healthy ageing as a public issue. Although there is not a clearly formulated policy on healthy ageing in the UK, there is a commitment to sustaining activity beyond employment, as stated in the Cabinet Office report, *Winning the Generation Game*. Thus, there are two elements to active ageing: (1) employment focused on the third age; and (2) healthy ageing and community participation targeted at the fourth age. Both have win–win potentials for older people and society in terms of social inclusion, well-being, QoL and in reducing pressures on public spending on pensions, health and social care (Walker 2002).

Third, there is globalization, which has exerted such a strong influence on policy discourses for the past five years or so (Held et al. 1999). In particular, there is the transatlantic consensus which holds, among other things, that globalization makes increasing inequality inevitable; global competition means taxation and social costs have to be minimized; and that traditional welfare states are not suited to a globalized world of differential lifecourses. The fact that older people are the main beneficiaries of welfare spending pushes pensions, health care and social care to the top of the reform agenda (Estes and Phillipson 2002; Walker and Deacon 2003).

Unlike some countries, the debate in the EU has not been purely about minimizing social costs, it is a twin-track one emphasizing prevention as well as remedial action. This starts from the assumption of individual responsibility but also includes recognition that the state has a crucial role in helping to establish the conditions within which people age. Put together, the policy line produced focused on extending activity and, with it, it is hoped, QoL. This tendency is reinforced by three subsidiary factors: the cultural shift towards individual QoL, usually labelled as late modernity or post-modernity. I mean the fact that people are ageing differently, experiencing ageing with diverse lifecourses and themselves seeking to enhance their own QoL. The mushrooming of pensioners' interest groups all over Europe in the past decade is one indicator of the new grassroots politics of old age which is impacting on the policy system (Walker and Naegele 1999; Estes et al. 2003). It is likely to increase when the 1960s baby boomers start to reach retirement around 2020. Then there is the traditional European social and political emphasis on solidarity and partnerships between state and citizen (Beck et al. 1997). Enhancing

QoL is an important element of this legacy and, at EU level, it figured as a goal of the Fifth Framework Research Programme while, in the UK, references to it can be found in countless documents such as the ESRC's priorities and the OST Foresight Panels' reports. Important policy developments such as the NHS Plan – the Performance Assessment framework and the 'best value' regime – and the National Service Frameworks all place a heavy emphasis on quality improvement. It is a major element of what the UK government and, increasingly the rest of the EU, calls 'modernization'.

Finally, there is the contribution of research itself to the emergence of ageing and QoL as major public issues. The UK's various scientific communities and their research councils have been very influential in raising the profile of both ageing and QoL research. There is a rich tradition of such research in the UK and other EU countries and, without it, extending quality life would not have been placed on the policy agenda so easily. For example, several of the key concepts being employed currently by policy-makers have been developed by and, therefore, gain their scientific legitimacy from, the discipline of social gerontology – the leading example being 'active ageing' itself.

The UK has some of the world's leading social gerontologists and their research has already contributed much to the quality of older people's lives. There are countless examples, from the impact of Peter Townsend's early work on both residential and home care to the series of studies by the late Tom Kitwood and his colleagues on ways to improve dementia care. This long research tradition has relied on researchers themselves taking the initiative and there has not been any attempt to 'join up' the various studies to see if, together, they reveal a more holistic picture of the quality of older people's lives. Nor, until recently, was there a concerted effort to encourage collaboration across the scientific disciplines yet, as everyone knows, ageing is not purely a social or a biological phenomenon. It is equally obvious that to improve the quality of older people's lives will require knowledge from a wide variety of different scientific disciplines – genetists, biologists, engineers, clinicians and social researchers. This realization dawned on the UK's scientific community later than its US counterpart. More precisely, the machinery to promote interdisciplinary collaboration was established in the USA much earlier than elsewhere. (The US Congress granted authority in 1974 to form the National Institute on Aging to provide leadership in ageing research, training, health information dissemination, and other programmes relevant to ageing and older people.) It was only in 2001 that four of the UK's research councils set up the National Collaboration on Ageing Research (NCAR) to promote interdisciplinary collaboration (http://www.shef.ac.uk/ukncar/). Then, from 2004, this innovation was replicated in several other EU countries under the European Research Area on Ageing Research (http://www.shef.ac.uk/era-age). In 2005 the four research councils behind the NCAR – the Economic and Social Research Council, the Engineering and Physical Sciences Research Council, the Basic and Biological Sciences Research Council and the Medical Research Council – launched a joint interdisciplinary research programme 'The New Dynamics of Ageing' (http://www.shef.ac.uk/newdynamics).

Connecting research and policy

Ageing is high on the agendas of both policy and research in the UK, the EU and other developed countries. During the first half of this century the most rapid ageing will occur in the less developed countries and, therefore, it is fast climbing their policy and research agendas, although their infrastructures on both fronts are often poorly developed too. The UN's Madrid Plan of Action on Ageing and the Research Agenda on Ageing for the Twenty-First Century both give priority to less developed countries (Sidorenko and Walker 2004). Despite this increasing priority for ageing and several progressive global actions, the relationship between research and policy is not well understood. Indeed, it can sometimes be a difficult and mutually dissatisfying relationship for both researchers and policy-makers.

The reasons for this are straightforward even if the solutions are not. Both sides often have unrealistic expectations of the other. On the one hand, research cannot always be delivered to meet the unpredictable timetables of policy-making or to answer specific questions in a direct way and, on the other, policy is rarely the single event that rational scientists imagine it to be. More commonly, it is a myriad of apparently disjointed actions that sometimes coalesce and are labelled in retrospect as decisions. Policy-making is rarely a sequential process with clearly defined stages. As Weiss (1980) showed, decisions are not made, they accrete. In a similar vein, Heclo and Rein (1980) have emphasized that policy is not made in a series of sequential steps starting with problem definition and leading to policy decision. All the elements in the process may be happening at once. In some cases the process may *begin* with a public statement or commitment, for example, from the Prime Minister, and only afterwards is the necessary support mobilized and the details of the policy worked out.

Thus, the common models of the relationship between research and policy give a wholly misleading impression of reality. The two most common models are the *rational* one, in which research generates knowledge which compels action, and the *engineering* model, in which it is policy that determines the demand for research (Booth 1988). In the former, the researcher is believed to influence policy while in the latter it is the policy-maker who sets the research questions. Both models are idealized versions of the policy-making process. Underlying both is a mistaken perception of policy-making as sequential and an over-emphasis on the role of research in this process.

In practice, research may have a number of different functions such as to legitimate policies, to vindicate the actions of policy-makers, as a mechanism of control and to provide symbolic value (what we might call, after Lipsky (1971) the MSG role – enhancing the colour and appearance rather than altering the substance). Policy-makers have other sources of information on which they draw and, often, all the sources are merged together. It must be remembered too that the policy process is political and, therefore, it entails struggles and compromises that may by-pass research evidence (Hill 1997). With regard to the world of practice, there are additional barriers to the effective utilization of research, such as forms of professional training that discourage openness to evidence, bureaucratic rules and stressful occupations that do not allow significant space to absorb new research findings. In fact, there are various different routes that can lead to policy without any recourse to evidence, such as improvisation or acting off the cuff, the repetition of recipes tried before in similar circumstances and as a result of unintended consequences of other actions (Weiss 1986). Very often policy, like 'stuff', just happens. This poses a tricky problem for research, as Booth (1988: 243) puts it:

> The absence of a single, authoritative policy maker, the elusiveness of decisions, and the twists and turns of the policy process have one important repercussion: they leave no obvious point of entry for research.

In these circumstances the relationship between research and policy is perhaps best seen as one that aspires to *enlightenment*. In other words, research is seldom used in a direct and instrumental way in the making of policy but, rather, it feeds into decision-making by a slow process of osmosis through which it may influence the thinking of policy-makers and help to frame their understanding of social reality and the possibilities for action. Thus, research may be as useful for its ideas as the specific data it generates. This means that a key challenge for researchers is to present findings in ways that are accessible for policy-makers and, ideally, at times when they need them, which in turn suggests the need for less strongly discipline-based research and more multi-disciplinary and policy-oriented research. Researchers have to see themselves as only one source of information for the policy process and not as having all the answers. For their part, policy-makers must be more open to the questions that research raises about practice and must engage in continuous dialogues with researchers.

It was in the light of this understanding of the complex, sometimes uneasy, relationship between research and the world of policy (including policy with regard to practice) that the GO Programme was oriented from the start towards an enlightenment approach. Thus, for example, the Programme sought to permeate the policy process at its pinnacle, in Whitehall, by connecting researchers with key policy-makers linked to the Inter-ministerial Committee on Older People. It produced a set of summary findings documents oriented towards the policy and practice communities, a specially commissioned booklet for policy-makers (Dean 2003) and arranged seminars between researchers and policy-makers. Despite these efforts there is no guarantee that the results of the GO Programme will be utilized. That is the nature of the relationship between research and policy: not exactly strangers but distant cousins that meet occasionally. Even in an era in which the case for evidence-based policy is frequently proclaimed, the inherently political character of policy-making means that unless researchers are deeply embedded within the ruling party or elite, they are unlikely to influence directly the outcome of decisions. Yet, in another version of Catch-22, if they do become partisan advocates of particular causes the validity of their research will be questioned and their status as scientists will be undermined by the political process in which they are embroiled.

While the likelihood of research directly affecting policy decisions is rare, its prospects with regard to practice are much rosier. In the UK there is increasing awareness of the need for health and social care service delivery to be evidence-based. This is reflected in the NHS in the importance of clinical governance and quality assessments by the Health Care Commission and in social care by the Social Institute for Excellence (SCIE). A very positive development for the GO Programme in this respect was the publication of the GO Findings series on the SCIE website.

Structure and agency in extending quality life

So far this chapter has focused exclusively on the research–policy relationship, which is its main intention, but it cannot be overlooked that ageing is a very personal issue as well. After all, it is older people who are living the extended years of life and, in doing so, who devise their own strategies or who respond to later life events as they happen. This raises the question about the respective roles of policy and individual action in determining QoL – a current controversy in social gerontology that continues the long-standing debate in sociology about the relationship between structure and ageing (Weber 1968; Archer 2000). The details of the current debate are discussed elsewhere (Walker 2005b) but, in essence, the political economy of ageing approach is criticized for neglecting agency (Gilleard and Higgs 2000). In fact, one of the key factors in the introduction of the political economy approach was the over-emphasis on agency in early social gerontology theorizing (Walker 1981). Rather than neglecting agency, it sought to show how its exercise is constrained by structures (which include policies). In other words, the ability of people to act within, engage with and change social structures is subject to conditions of relative power and powerlessness. It hardly needs stressing that, on average, older people from professional and managerial occupations have more chances to construct and elaborate their own unique pattern of responses to ageing than do those from semi-skilled and unskilled ones. Similarly, older women and ethnic minority elders experience poverty and social exclusion – two heavy constraints on agency – at higher rates than men and the white majority. Political economy theory, in a nutshell, is concerned with the distribution of power and, therefore, it must encompass the relationships in which power is exercised, in short, both agency and structure. The notion that it is possible to choose between agency and identity and structural location and influence is false (Gilleard and Higgs 2000: 12). In practice, individual ageing is determined by the interaction between social actors and social structures. The practical gerontological importance of this constant tension between agency and structure is that the experience of ageing, including its quality, is the result of a combination of structural elements, such as social class, income, wealth, gender and ethnicity, and individual actions and choices. This can be illustrated from the GO Programme research reported in this book.

For example, Arber and colleagues (2003a) show the disadvantage experienced by divorced women and widows compared with married men: at work here are aspects of both structure (for example, gender, employment, occupational pensions and social security) and agency (for example, marriage, divisions of domestic labour and household finances). Breeze and her co-researchers (2002) demonstrate the clear social class gradient in functional limitation and reported problems with self-care, with the most disadvantaged group being those in social classes IV or V living in council or housing association accommodation. In this example, agency in terms of mobility to get around and care for oneself is directly constrained by structure. Both these examples are summarized in Chapter 3. In the same chapter the results of the research by Nazroo and his colleagues (2003) show the substantial inequalities in QoL between ethnic minority older people and their white counterparts, as well as between these groups, for example, with regard to incomes. At the same time the important finding from this project that ethnic minority older people derive higher QoL from their (often deprived) neighbourhoods than do the majority white population suggests that agency is being exercised effectively to some extent within a structure of inequality. Evandrou and Glaser (2002a) reinforce this picture of structural constraints on agency with reference to the relative disadvantage in the pension system experienced by women who have carried multiple role responsibilities in mid-life (Chapter 5). The policy implications of this body of research focusing on inequalities and structural constraints are straightforward, if not politically feasible. They include the raising of basic state pension levels, improved pension protection for people providing care, action to combat various kinds of discrimination in the labour and housing market and measures (such as taxation) aimed at reducing income inequalities.

Some GO projects focused on individual adaptation to ageing, for example, among frail older people (Chapter 8). This work reveals discontinuities in personal identity resulting from later life losses, such as one's home and friends, and a decline in physical health or cognitive functioning. Those in a residential setting may feel particularly cut off from their previous lives. At the same time, in the face of overwhelming structural constraints, frail older people often attempt to maintain their identity by, for instance, trying to have a significant role in the family and keeping active in mind and body. Baldock and Hadlow's (2002) research revealed the extraordinary lengths that frail housebound older people can go to in exercising identity-protecting agency by rejecting services. Communication plays a key role in this exercise of agency to maintain identity, through building relationships and sustaining friendships, and through participation in meaningful activities. Interaction and communication are essential to agency. The projects that focused on maintaining identity in the face of frailty point to policy changes aimed at enhancing individual agency. In particular, they contain important messages for practitioners working with such older people, including the role of reminiscence (McKee et al. 2002) and the need for rapid interventions to maintain social contacts following the onset of severe disability (Baldock and Hadlow 2002).

Thus, the GO Programme provides ample proof that QoL in old age is the product of the inter-relationship between structure and agency over the lifecourse. This is powerfully evinced in the work of Bowling and her colleagues (2002) which combined data from a major nationally representative quantitative survey and in-depth follow-up interviews (Chapter 2) to formulate the foundations for a good QoL in old age:

- having good social relationships with family, friends and neighbours;

- having social roles and participating in social and voluntary activities, plus other activities/hobbies performed alone;

- having good health and functional ability;

- living in a good home and good neighbourhood;

- having a positive outlook and psychological well-being;

- having adequate income;

- maintaining independence and control over one's life.

Mainly these foundations of a good QoL contain a mixture of factors reflecting both structure and agency and their combination. Thus, the policy prescriptions aimed at extending QoL which arise from this work, as for the GO Programme as a whole, must contain a mixture of those aimed, on the one hand, at reducing disadvantages and inequalities that constrain action and, on the other, at promoting self-efficacy and self-realization and the maintenance of health and capacity. In other words, policies to extend quality life must address both structure and agency and, ideally, in a mutually reinforcing way.

As to the precise focus of policy and interventions, Chapter 3 reports on the project by Blane and colleagues (2002) which found that contemporary factors had a greater impact on QoL than lifecourse ones. However, they also note the implicit influence of lifecourse factors in many contemporary ones, including pensions, health and friendships. Thus, a strategy to promote QoL in old age should include policies aimed at the lifecourse, such as active ageing, and those directed mainly at older people (a distinction that in the Madrid Plan of Action on Ageing is labelled ageing mainstreaming and ageing specific).

The important policy point to end with is that the GO Programme provides the evidence base on which a strategy to extend quality life could be based. The big changes that are required, ultimately, are a matter of political commitment, but also there is a myriad of small, relatively inexpensive, innovations in policy and practice that could be made quickly and which would immediately improve older people's lives. There are also steps that older people themselves may take without reference to policy and practice. The most effective way forward is likely to be a combination of individual action, practice innovations and policy development, but older people themselves must be integral to structural changes if these are to enhance older people's own capacity to enjoy lives of quality.

References

Abramson, L.Y., Matalsky, G.I. and Alloy, L.B. (1989) Hopelessness depression: a theory-based subtype of depression, *Psychological Review*, 96: 358–72.

Adelman, P.K. (1994a) Multiple roles and psychological well-being in a national sample of older adults, *Journal of Gerontology: Social Sciences*, 49: S277–85.

Adelman, P.K. (1994b) Multiple roles and physical health among older adults, *Research on Aging*, 16: 142–66.

Afshar, H., Franks, M. and Maynard, M. (2002) *Women, Ethnicity and Empowerment in Later Life*. GO Findings 10, Sheffield: Growing Older Programme, University of Sheffield.

Ahmad, W.I.U. (2000) Introduction, in W.I.U. Ahmad (ed.) *Ethnicity, Disability and Chronic Illness*. Buckingham: Open University Press: 1–11.

Ahmad, W.I.U. and Atkin, K. (1996) *'Race' and Community Care*. Buckingham: Open University Press.

Ainley, S.C., Singleton Jr, J. and Swigert, V. (1992) Aging and religious participation: reconsidering the effects of health, *Journal for the Scientific Study of Religion*, 31(2): 175–88.

Aldous, J. (1995) New views of grandparents in intergenerational context, *Journal of Family Issues*, 16(1): 104–22.

Anderson, R. (1988) The contribution of informal care to the management of stroke, *International Disability Studies*, 10(3): 107–12.

Andersson, L. (1998) Loneliness research and interventions: a review of the literature, *Ageing and Mental Health*, 2(4): 264–74.

Andrews, F.M. and Withey, S.B. (1976) *Social Indicators of Well Being: Americans' Perceptions of Life Quality*. New York: Plenum.

Aquino, J.A., Russell, D.W., Cutrona, C.E. and Altmaier, E.M. (1996) Employment status, social support and life satisfaction among the elderly, *Journal of Counselling Psychology*, 43: 480–9.

Arber, S., Davidson, K., Daly, T. and Perren, K. (2003) *Older Men: Their Social Worlds and Healthy Lifestyles*. GO Findings 12, Sheffield: Growing Older Programme, University of Sheffield.

Arber, S. and Evandrou, M. (1993) Mapping the territory: ageing, independence and the life course, in S. Arber and M. Evandrou (eds) *Ageing, Independence and the Life Course*. London: Jessica Kingsley: 9–26.

Arber, S. and Ginn, J. (1991) *Gender and Later Life: A Sociological Analysis of Resources and Constraints*. London: Sage.

Arber, S. and Ginn, J. (eds) (1995) *Connecting Gender and Ageing*. Buckingham: Open University Press.

Arber, S. and Ginn, J. (2004) Ageing and gender: diversity and change, *Social Trends 2004 Edition, No. 34*. Office for National Statistics, London: The Stationery Office.

Arber, S., Price, D., Davidson, K. and Perren, K. (2003) Re-examining gender and marital status: material well-being and social involvement in later life, in S. Arber, K. Davidson and J. Ginn (eds) *Gender and Ageing: Changing Roles and Relationships*. Maidenhead: Open University Press: 148–67.

Archer, M. (2000) *Being Human: The Problem of Agency*, Cambridge: Cambridge University Press.

Aronson, M.K. and Lipkowitz, R. (1981) Senile dementia, Alzheimer's type: the family and the health care delivery system, *Journal of the American Geriatrics Society*, 29: 568–71.

Ayis, S., Gooberman-Hill, R. and Ebrahim, S. (2003) Long-standing and limiting illness in older people: associations with chronic diseases, psychosocial and environmental factors, *Age and Ageing*, 32(3): 265–72.

Bajekal, M., Blane, D., Grewal, I., Karlsen, S. and Nazroo, J. (2004) Ethnic differences in influences on quality of life at older ages: a quantitative analysis, *Ageing and Society*, 24: 709–728.

Baldock, J. and Hadlow, J. (2002) *Housebound Older People: The Links between Identity, Self-Esteem and the Use of Care Services*. GO Findings 4, Sheffield: Growing Older Programme, University of Sheffield.

Baldock, J. and Ungerson, C. (1994) *Becoming Consumers of Community Care: Households within the Mixed Economy of Care*. York: Joseph Rowntree Foundation.

Ball, K., Berch, D.B., Helmers, K.F. et al. (2002) Effects of cognitive training interventions with older adults: a randomised control trial, *Journal of the American Medical Association*, 288: 2271–81.

Baltes, P.B. and Baltes, M.M. (1990) Psychological perspectives on successful aging: the model of selective optimization with compensation, in P.B. Baltes and M.M. Baltes (eds) *Successful Aging: Perspectives from the Behavioral Sciences*. New York: Cambridge University Press: 1–34.

Barnes, M. and Warren, L. (eds) (1999) *Paths to Empowerment*. Bristol: The Policy Press.

Barrow, G.M. (1992), *Aging, the Individual and Society*, 5th edn. St Paul, MN: West Publishing Company.

Bartley, M., Popay, J. and Plewis, I. (1992) Domestic conditions, paid employment and women's experience of ill-health, *Sociology of Health & Illness*, 14: 313–43.

Bauman, Z. (1999) *Work, Consumerism and the New Poor*. Buckingham: Open University Press.

Beaumont, J.G. and Kenealy, P. (2003) *Quality of Life of Healthy Older People: Residential Setting and Social Comparison Processes*. Growing Older Findings 20, Growing Older Programme, University of Sheffield, Sheffield.

Beaumont, J.G., Kenealy, P.M. and Murrell, R.C. (2003) *Quality of Life (QoL) of the Healthy Elderly: Residential Setting and Social Comparison Processes*. End of Award Report on Project L480254002 to the Economic and Social Research Council. www.regard.ac.uk

Beck, B., Dallinger, U., Naegele, G. and Reichert, M. (1997) *Vereinbarkeit von Erwerbstätigkeit und Pflege* [Balancing Work and Elder Care]. Stuttgart: Kohlhammer.

Beck, U. (1992) *Risk Society*. London: Sage.

Beck, W., van der Maesen, L. and Walker, A. (1997) *The Social Quality of Europe*. London: Kluwer Law International.

Benner, P. (1985) Quality of life: a phenomenological perspective on explanation, prediction and understanding in nursing science, *Advances in Nursing Science: Special Issue: Quality of Life*, 8: 1–14.

Bennett, K.M. and Bennett, G. (2000–2001) 'And there's always this great hole inside that hurts': an empirical study of bereavement in later life, *Omega*, 42(3): 237–51.

Bennett, K.M., Hughes, G.M. and Smith, P.T 'This is me': Augmented identity and the transition from married to widowed status in older women (submitted).

Bennett, K.M. and Vidal-Hall, S. (2000) Narratives of death: a qualitative study of widowhood in later life, *Ageing and Society*, 20: 413–28.

Berghman, J. (1997) The resurgence of poverty and the struggle against exclusion: a new challenge for social security?, *International Social Security Review*, 50(1): 3–23.

Bergner, M., Bobbitt, R.A., Carter, W.B. and Gilson, B.S. (1981) The Sickness Impact Profile: development and final revision of a health status measure, *Medical Care*, XIX: 787–805.

Bernard, M. (2000) *Promoting Health in Old Age*. Buckingham: Open University Press.

Berney, L. and Blane, D. (1997) Collecting retrospective data: accuracy of recall after 50 years judged against historical records, *Social Science and Medicine*, 45: 1519–25.

Biggs, S. (1993) *Understanding Ageing: Images, Attitudes and Professional Practice*. Buckingham: Open University Press.

Biggs, S. (1997) Choosing not to be old? Masks, bodies and identity management in later life, *Ageing and Society*, 17(5): 553–70.

Biggs, S. (2004) Age, gender, narratives and masquerades, *Journal of Aging Studies*, 18(1): 45–58.

Blakemore, K. and Boneham, M. (1994) *Age, Race and Ethnicity: A Comparative Approach*. Buckingham: Open University Press.

Blane, D. (1999) The life course, the social gradient and health, in M. Marmot and R.G. Wilkinson (eds) *Social Determinants of Health*. Oxford: Oxford University Press: 64–80.

Blane, D., Bartley, M. and Davey Smith, G. (1997) Disease aetiology and materialist explanations of socioeconomic mortality differentials, *European Journal of Public Health*, 7: 385–91.

Blane, D., Berney, L., Davey Smith, G., Gunnell, D. and Holland, P. (1999) Reconstructing the life course: a 60 year follow-up study based on the Boyd Orr cohort, *Public Health*, 113: 117–24.

Blane, D., Higgs, P., Hyde, M. and Wiggins, R. (2004) Life course influences on quality of life in early old age, *Social Science and Medicine*, 58: 2171–9.

Blane, D., Wiggins, R., Higgs, P. and Hyde, M. (2002) *Inequalities in Quality of Life in Early Old Age*. GO Findings 9, Sheffield: Growing Older Programme, University of Sheffield.

Booth, T. (1988) *Developing Policy Research*. Aldershot: Avebury.

Bourdieu, P. (1984) *Distinction: A Social Critique of the Judgement of Taste*. Cambridge, MA: Harvard University Press.

Bowlby, J. (1981) *Attachment and Loss*, Vol. 3: *Loss, Sadness and Depression*. Harmondsworth: Penguin.

Bowling, A. (1995) The most important things in life: comparisons between older and younger population age group by gender. Results from a national survey of the public's judgements, *International Journal of Health Science*, 6(4): 160–75.

Bowling, A. (1997) *Measuring Health: A Review of Quality of Life Measurement Scales*, 2nd edn. Maidenhead: Open University Press.

Bowling, A., Banister, D., Sutton, S., Evans, O. and Windsor, J. (2002a) A multidimensional model of the quality of life in older age, *Aging and Mental Health*, 6(4): 355–71.

Bowling, A., Farquhar, M. and Browne, P. (1991) Life satisfaction and associations with social networks and support variables in three samples of elderly people, *International Journal of Geriatric Psychiatry*, 6: 549–66.

Bowling, A. and Gabriel, Z. (2004). An integrational model of quality of life in older age: a comparison of analytic and lay models of quality of life, *Social Indicators Research*, 69: 1–36.

Bowling, A., Gabriel, Z., Banister, D. and Sutton, S. (2002b) *Adding Quality to Quantity: Older People's Views on their Quality of Life and Its Enhancement*. GO Findings 7, Sheffield: Growing Older Programme, University of Sheffield.

Bowling, A., Sutton, S.R. and Banister, D. (2003) *Adding Quality to Quantity: Older People's Views on their Quality of Life and Its Enhancement*. Final report on ESRC grant number L 480254003. http://www.regard.ac.uk/research_findings/L480254003/report.pdf

Brandstädter, J. and Renner, G. (1990) Tenacious goal pursuit and flexible goal adjustment: explication and age-related analysis of assimilative and accommodative strategies of coping *Psychology of Aging* 5: 58–67.

Braun, M.J. and Berg, D.H. (1994) Meaning reconstruction in the experience of parental bereavement, *Death Studies*, 18: 105–29.

Breeze, E., Grundy, C., Fletcher, A., Wilkinson, P., Jones, D. and Bulpitt, C. (2002) *Inequalities in Quality of Life Among People Aged 75 Years and Over in*

Great Britain. GO Findings 1, Sheffield: Growing Older Programme, University of Sheffield.

Brooker, D. (forthcoming) What is person-centred care? *Reviews in Clinical Gerontology*.

Brooker, D. and Duce, L. (2000) Wellbeing and activity in dementia: a comparison of group reminiscence therapy, structured goal-directed group activity and unstructured time. *Aging and Mental Health*, 4: 354–8.

Bruce, E., Surr, C. and Tibbs, M.A. (2002) *A Special Kind of Care: Improving Well-Being in People Living with Dementia*. Final report to Methodist Home Care Group. http://www.brad.ac.uk/acad/health/bdg/research/methodist.php

Burchardt, T., Le Grand, J. and Piachaud, D. (1999) Social exclusion in Britain 1991–1995, *Social Policy and Administration*, 33(3): 227–44.

Burnett, J.J. (1991) Examining the media habits of the affluent elderly, *Journal of Advertising Research*, October: 33–41.

Butt, J. and Mirza, K. (1996) *Social Care and Black Communities*. London: HMSO.

Bytheway, B. and Johnson, J. (1998) The site of age, in S. Nettleton and J. Watson (eds) *The Body in Everyday Life*. London: Routledge: 243–57.

Calasanti, T. (1996) Incorporating diversity: meaning, levels of research and implications for theory, *Gerontologist*, 36(2): 147–56.

Calasanti, T. (2004) New directions in feminist gerontology: an introduction, *Journal of Aging Studies*, 18(1): 1–8.

Calasanti, T. and Slevin, K. (2001) *Gender, Social Inequalities and Aging*. Walnut Creek, CA: AltaMira Press.

Campbell, A. (1981) *The Sense of Well-Being in America*. New York: McGraw-Hill.

Cantor, N. and Sanderson, C.A. (1999) Life task participation and well-being: the importance of taking part in daily life, in D. Kahneman, E. Diener and N. Schwarz (eds) *Well-Being: The Foundations of Hedonic Psychology*. New York: Russell Sage Foundation: 230–43.

Carstensen, L.L., Gross, J.J. and Fung, H.H. (1997) The social context of emotional experience, *Annual Review of Gerontology and Geriatrics*, 17: 325–52.

Casper, L.M. and Bryson, K.R. (1998) Co-resident grandparents and their grandchildren: grandparent-maintained families. Paper presented to the Population Association of America Conference, March 2000, Los Angeles.

Cattell, V. and Evans, M. (1999) *Neighbourhood Images in East London: Social Capital and Social Networks on Two East London Estates*. York: Joseph Rowntree Foundation, YPS.

Chambers Twentieth Century Dictionary, rev. edn. (1961) Edinburgh: W. and R. Chambers.

Chiverton, P. and Caine, E.D. (1989) Education to assist spouses in coping with Alzheimer's disease: a controlled trial, *Journal of the American Geriatrics Society*, 37: 539–98.

Chung, M.C., Killingworth, A. and Nolan, P. (1997) A critique of the concept of quality of life, *International Journal of Health Care Quality Assurance*, 10(2): 80–4.

Clarke, L. and Roberts, C. (2003) *Grandparenthood: its Meaning and its Contribution to Older People's Lives*. ESRC Growing Older Programme Research Findings No. 22, Sheffield: University of Sheffield.

Cobb, A.K. and Forbes, S. (2002) Qualitative research? What does it have to offer to the gerontologist? *Journals of Gerontology*, 57: M197–M202.

Coleman, P.G. (1984) Assessing self-esteem and its sources in elderly people, *Ageing and Society*, 4(2): 117–35.

Coleman, P.G., Ivani-Chalian, C. and Robinson, M. (2004) Religious attitudes among British older people: stability and change in a 20 year longitudinal study, *Ageing and Society*, 24: 167–88.

Coleman, P.G., Ivani-Chalian, C. and Robinson, M. (1993) Self-esteem and its sources; stability and change in later life, *Ageing and Society*, 13(3): 171–92.

Coleman, P.G., McKiernan, F., Mills, M.A. and Speck, P. (2002) Spiritual belief and quality of life: the experience of older bereaved spouses, *Quality in Ageing, Policy, Practice and Research*, 3: 20–6.

Cook, J., Maltby, T. and Warren, L. (2003) *Older Women's Lives and Voices: Participation and Policy in Sheffield*. GO Findings 21, Sheffield: Growing Older Programme, University of Sheffield.

Cook, J., Maltby, T. and Warren, L. (2004) A participatory approach to older women's quality of life, in A. Walker and C. Hagan Hennessey (eds) *Growing Older: Quality of Life in Old Age*. Maidenhead: Open University Press: 149–66.

Coulthard, M., Walker, A. and Morgan, A. (2002) *People's Perceptions of their Neighborhood and Community Involvement: Results from the Social Capital Module of the General Household Survey 2000*. London: The Stationery Office.

Craig, G. (2004) Citizenship, exclusion and older people, *Journal of Social Policy*, 33: 95–114.

Cully, J.A., LaVoie, D. and Gfeller, J.D. (2001) Reminiscence, personality and psychological functioning in older adults. *The Gerontologist*, 41: 89–95.

Dannefer, D. (2003) Cumulative advantage/disadvantage and the life course: Cross-fertilizing age and social science theory, *Journals of Gerontology B Series: Social Sciences*, 53: S327–37.

Dautzenberg, M., Diederiks, J.P.M., Philipsen, H. and Stevens, F. (1998) Women of a middle generation and parent care, *International Journal of Aging and Human Development*, 47: 241–62.

Davidson, K. and Arber, S. (2004) Older men, their health behaviours and partnership status, in A. Walker and C. Hagan Hennessy (eds) *Growing Older: Quality of Life in Old Age*. Maidenhead: Open University Press: 127–48.

Davidson, K., Daly, T. and Arber, S. (2003) Exploring the worlds of older men, in S. Arber, K. Davidson and J. Ginn (eds) *Gender and Ageing: Changing Roles and Relationships*. Maidenhead: Open University Press/McGraw-Hill: 168–85.

Dean, M. (2003) *Growing Older in the 21st Century*. Swindon: ESRC.

de Jong Gierveld, J. (1987) Developing and testing a model of loneliness, *Journal of Personal and Social Psychology*, 53: 119–28.

de Jong Gierveld, J. (1998) A review of loneliness: concepts and definitions, causes and consequences, *Reviews in Clinical Gerontology*, 8: 73–80.

de Jong Gierveld, J. and Kamphuis, F. (1985) The development of a Rasch-type loneliness scale, *Applied Psychological Measurement*, 9(3): 289–99.

DeMaio, T.J. (1984) Social desirability and survey measurement: a review, in C.F. Turner and E. Martin (eds) *Surveying Subjective Phenomena*, Vol. 2. New York: Russell Sage Foundation.

Department for Education and Employment (DfEE) (2000) *Changing Patterns in a Changing World*. Edinburgh: DfEE and The Scottish Office.

Department of the Environment, Transport and the Regions (1998) *English House Condition Survey 1996*. London: The Stationery Office.

Department of Health (2003) *Direct Payments Guidance Community Care, Services for Carers and Children's Services (Direct Payments) Guidance England 2003*. London: Department of Health.

Department for Work and Pensions (2002) *Households Below Average Income.* London: Department for Work and Pensions.

Department for Work and Pensions (2003) *The Pensioners' Incomes Series, 2001/2*, Pensions Analysts Division. London: The Stationery Office.

DETR (1998) *Updating and Revising the Index of Local Deprivation.* London: Department of the Environment, Transport and the Regions. London: The Stationery Office.

Diener, E. (1984) Subjective well-being, *Psychological Bulletin*, 235: 542–75.

Diener, E. (2000) Subjective well-being: the science of happiness and a proposal for a national index, in M.E.P. Seligman and M. Csikszentmihalyi (eds) *Special Issue on Happiness, Excellence and Optimal Human Functioning. American Psychologist*, 55, January: 34–43.

Diener, E. and Lucas, R.E. (1999) Personality and subjective well-being, in D. Kahneman, E. Diener and N. Schwarz (eds) *Well-Being: The Foundations of Hedonic Psychology.* New York: Russell Sage Foundation: 13–229.

Doka, K.J. (1989) *Disenfranchised Grief: Recognizing Hidden Sorrow.* San Francisco: Jossey-Bass.

Donne, J. (1990) *John Donne*, ed. John Carey. Oxford: Oxford University Press.

Dowd, J. (1980) *Stratification Among the Aged.* Monterey, CA: Brooks/Cole.

Dowswell, G., Lawler, J., Dowswell, T., Young, J., Forster, A. and Hearn, J. (2000) Investigating recovery from stroke: a qualitative study, *Journal of Clinical Nursing*, 9(4): 507–15.

Doyal, L. and Gough, I. (1991) *A Theory of Human Need.* London: Macmillan.

Dressel, P., Minkler, M. and Yen, I. (1998) Gender, race, class and aging: advances and opportunities, in M. Minkler and C.L. Estes (eds) *Critical Gerontology: Perspectives from Political and Moral Economy.* Amityville, NY: Baywood Publishing Company, Inc: 275–94.

Drew, L.A. (2000) Grandparents and divorce, *Journal of the British Society of Gerontology*, 10(3): 7–10.

Eaves, Y.D. (2000) 'What happened to me': rural African American elders' experiences of stroke, *Journal of Neuroscience Nursing*, 32(1): 37–48.

Elder, G.H. (1974) *Children of the Great Depression.* Chicago: University of Chicago Press.

Ellis-Hill, C., Payne, S. and Ward, C. (2000) Self-body split: issues of identity in physical recovery after stroke, *Disability and Rehabilitation*, 22(16): 725–33.

Erikson, E.H., Erikson, J.M. and Kivnick, H.Q. (1986) *Vital Involvement in Old Age*. London: W.W. Norton.

Estes, C., Biggs, S. and Phillipson, C. (2003) *Social Theory, Social Policy and Ageing: A Critical Introduction*. Maidenhead: Open University Press.

Estes, C. and Phillipson, C. (2002) The globalisation of capital, the welfare state and old age policy, *International Journal of Health Services*, 32(2): 279–97.

Evandrou, M. and Glaser, K. (2002a) *Family, Work and Quality of Life: Changing Economic and Social Roles*. GO Findings 5, Sheffield: Growing Older Programme, University of Sheffield.

Evandrou, M. and Glaser, K. (2002b) Changing economic and social roles: the experience of four cohorts of mid-life individuals in Britain, 1985–2000, *Population Trends*, 110: 19–30.

Evandrou, M. and Glaser, K. (2003) Combining work and family life: the pension penalty of caring, *Ageing and Society*, 23: 583–601.

Evandrou, M., Glaser, K. and Henz, U. (2002) Multiple role occupancy in mid-life: balancing work and family life in Britain, *The Gerontologist*, 42(6): 781–89.

Farkas, J.I. and Himes, C.L. (1997) The influence of caregiving and employment on the voluntary activities of midlife and older women, *Journal of Gerontology: Social Sciences*, 52B: S180–9.

Farquhar, M. (1995) Elderly people's definitions of quality of life, *Social Science and Medicine*, 41: 1439–46.

Featherstone, M. and Hepworth, M. (1991) The mask of ageing and the postmodern life course, in M. Featherstone, M. Hepworth and B.S. Turner (eds) *The Body: Social Process and Cultural Theory*. London: Sage: 371–89.

Featherstone, M. and Hepworth, M. (1993) Images of ageing, in J. Bond, P. Coleman and S. Peace (eds) *Ageing in Society: An Introduction to Social Gerontology*. London: Sage.

Ferguson, N. with Douglas, G., Lowe, N., Murch, M. and Robinson, M. (2004) *Grandparenting in Divorced Families*. Bristol: Policy Press.

Fielding, N. and Fielding, J. (1986) *Linking Data: The Articulation of Qualitative and Quantitative Methods in Social Research*. London: Sage.

Finch, J. (1989) *Family Obligations and Social Change*. Cambridge: Polity Press.

Fletcher, A., Jones, D., Bulpitt, C. and Tulloch, A. (2002) The MRC trial of assessment and management of older people in the community: objectives, design and interventions [ISRCTN23494848], *BMC Health Services Research*, 2(1): 21.

Fournier, S. and Fine, G. (1990) Jumping grannies: exercise as a buffer against becoming old. *Play and Culture* 3: 337–342.

Friedman, M. (1997) Autonomy and social relationships: rethinking the feminist critique, in D. Tietjens Meyers (ed.) *Feminists Rethink the Self*. Oxford: Westview Press.

Fry, P.S. (1998) Spousal loss in late life: a 1-year follow-up of perceived changes in life meaning and psychological functioning following bereavement, *Journal of Personal and Interpersonal Loss*, 3: 369–91.

Fuller-Thompson, E., Minkler, M. and Driver, D. (1997) A profile of grandparents raising grandchildren in the United States, *The Gerontologist*, 37(3): 406–11.

Gabriel, Z. and Bowling, A. (2004) Quality of life in old age from the perspectives of older people, in A. Walker and C.H. Hennessy (eds) *Growing Older: Quality of Life in Old Age*. Maidenhead: Open University Press: 14–34.

Giddens, A. (1994) *Beyond Left and Right*. Cambridge: Polity Press.

Gilhooly, K., Gilhooly, M., Phillips, L. and Hanlon, P. (2003). Use it or lose it? cognitive functioning in older adults. *Nursing and Residential Care*, 5(8): 392–5.

Gilhooly, M. (2001) Quality of life and real life cognitive functioning, *Growing Older Programme Newsletter*, 2: 6.

Gilhooly, M., Hamilton, K., O'Neill, M., Gow, J., Webster, N. and Pike, F. (2003) *Transport and Ageing: Extending Quality of Life via Public and Private Transport*. GO Findings 16, Sheffield: Growing Older Programme, University of Sheffield.

Gilhooly, M., Phillips, L., Gilhooly, K. and Hanlon, P. (2003) *Quality of Life and Real Life Cognitive Functioning*. GO Findings 15, Sheffield: Growing Older Programme, University of Sheffield.

Gilhooly, M., Phillips, L., Gilhooly, K. et al. (2002b) *Quality of Life and Real Life Cognitive Functioning*. End of award report on ESRC Award Reference Number L480 25 40 29.

Gilhooly, M.L.M., Zarit, S.H. and Birren, J.E. (1986) *The Dementias: Policy and Management*. Englewood Cliffs, NJ: Prentice Hall.

Gill, T.M. and Feinstein, A.R. (1994) A critical appraisal of the quality of life measurements, *Journal of the American Medical Association*, 272: 619–26.

Gilleard, C. and Higgs, P. (2000) *Cultures of Ageing: Self, Citizen and the Body*. Harlow: Prentice Hall.

Gilleard, C. and Higgs, P. (2002) The third age: class, cohort or generation?, *Ageing and Society* 22: 369–82.

Ginn, J. (2003) *Gender, Pensions and the Lifecourse: How Pensions Need to Adapt to Changing Family Forms*. Bristol: Policy Press.

Ginn, J., Street, D. and Arber, S. (eds) (2001) *Women, Work and Pensions*. Buckingham: Open University Press.

Gjonça, E. and Calderwood, L. (2003) Methodology, in M. Marmot, J. Banks, R. Blundell, C. Lessof and J. Nazroo (eds) *Health, Wealth and Lifestyles of the Older Population in England: The 2002 English Longitudinal Study of Ageing*. London: IFS.

Glass, T.A., Mendes de Leon, C., Marottoli, R.A. et al. (1999) Population based study of social and productive activities as predictors of survival among elderly Americans. *British Medical Journal* 319: 478–83.

Goffman, E. (1963) *Stigma: Notes on the Management of Spoiled Identity*. Englewood Cliffs, NJ: Prentice Hall.

Gold, D.P., Andres, D., Etezadi, K. et al. (1995) Structural equation model of intellectual change and continuity and predictors of intelligence in older men. *Psychology and Aging*, 10: 294–303.

Goldberg, D. (1978) *Manual of the General Health Questionnaire*. Windsor: NFER-Nelson.

Goldberg, D. and Williams, P. (1988) *A User's Guide to the General Health Questionnaire*. Windsor: The NFER-Nelson Publishing Company Limited.

Goode, W. (1960) A theory of role strain, *American Sociological Review*, 25: 483–96.

Gordon, D. et al. (2000) *Poverty and Social Exclusion in Britain*. York: Joseph Rowntree Foundation.

Gorer, G. (1965) *Death, Grief and Mourning in Contemporary Britain*. London: Tavistock.

Graham, H. (2002) Building an inter-disciplinary science of health inequalities: the example of life course research, *Social Science and Medicine*, 55: 2005–16.

Granger, C.V., Albrecht, G.L. and Hamilton, B.B. (1979) Outcome of comprehensive medical rehabilitation: measurement by PULSES profile and the Barthel Index, *Archives of Physical Medicine and Rehabilitation*, 60(4): 145–54.

Grant, J.S. (1996) Home care problems experienced by stroke survivors and their family caregivers, *Home Healthcare Nurse*, 14(11): 892–902.

Grewal, I., Nazroo, J., Bajekal, M., Blane, D. and Lewis, J. (2004) Influences on quality of life: a qualitative investigation of ethnic differences among older people in England, *Journal of Ethnic and Migration Studies* (in press).

Guillemard, A.-M. (ed.) (1984) *Old Age and the Welfare State*. New York: Sage.

Hambrick, D.Z., Salthouse, T.A. and Meinz, E.J. (1999) Predictors of crossword puzzle proficiency and moderators of age-cognition relations, *Journal of Experimental Psychology: General*, 12: 131–64.

Hart, E. (2001) System-induced setbacks in stroke recovery, *Sociology of Health and Illness*, 23(1): 101–23.

Heclo, H. and Rein, M. (1980) Social science and negative income taxation, in OECD, *The Utilisation of the Social Sciences in Policy Making in the US*. Paris: OECD.

Held, D., McGrew, A., Goldblatt, D. and Perraton, J. (1999) *Global Transformations: Politics, Economics and Culture*. Cambridge: Polity Press.

Hennessy, C.H. and Hennessy, M. (1990) Community-based long-term care for the elderly: evaluation practice reconsidered, *Medical Care Review*, 47: 221–59.

Hermans, H.J.M., Kempen, H.J.G. and van Loon, R.J.P. (1992) The dialogical self: beyond individualism and rationalism, *American Psychologist*, 47: 23–33.

Higgs, P., Hyde, M., Wiggins, R. and Blane, D. (2003) Researching quality of life in early old age: the importance of the sociological dimension, *Social Policy and Administration*, 37: 239–52.

Hill, M. (1997) *The Policy Process in the Modern State*, 3rd edn. Hemel Hempstead: Prentice Hall.

Hills, J. (1995) The welfare state and redistribution between generations, in J. Falkingham and J. Hills (eds) *The Dynamic of Welfare: The Welfare State and the Life Cycle*. Hemel Hempstead: Prentice Hall/Harvester Wheatsheaf.

Hinton, J. (1967) *Dying*. Harmondsworth: Penguin.

Hirsch, D. (2000) *Life after 50: Issues for Policy and Research*. York: YPS.

Hochschild, A.R. (1979) Emotion work, feeling rules and social support, *American Journal of Sociology*, 85: 551–73.

Holmen, K., Ericsson, K., Andersson, L. and Winblad, B. (1992) Loneliness among elderly people in Stockholm: a population study, *Journal of Advanced Nursing*, 17: 43–51.

Holmen, K., Ericsson, K., Andersson, L. and Winblad, B. (1994) Loneliness and living conditions of the oldest old, *Scandinavian Journal of Social Medicine*, 22: 15–19.

Holmen, K. and Furukawa, H. (2002) Loneliness, health and social network among elderly people: a follow-up study, *Archives of Gerontology and Geriatrics*, 35(3): 261–71.

Home Office (1998) *Supporting Families: A Consultation Document*. London: The Stationery Office.

Howse, K. (1999) *Religion and Spirituality in Later Life: A Review*. London: Centre for Policy on Ageing.

Hsieh, H.F. and Wang, J.J. (2003) Effect of reminiscence therapy on depression in older adults: a systematic review, *International Journal of Nursing Studies*, 40: 335–45.

Hubbard, G., Cook, A., Tester, S. et al. (2002) Beyond words: older people with dementia using and interpreting non-verbal behaviour, *Journal of Aging Studies*, 16(2): 155–67.

Hubbard, G., Tester, S. and Downs, M. (2003) Meaningful social interactions between older people in institutional care settings, *Ageing and Society*, 23(1): 99–114.

Hyde, M., Blane, D., Higgs, P. and Wiggins, R. (2001) The theory and properties of a needs satisfaction model of quality of life, *Growing Older Programme Newsletter*, 3: 4.

Hyde, M. and Janevic, M. (2003) Social activity, in M. Marmot, J. Banks, R. Blundell, C. Lessof and J. Nazroo (eds) *Health, Wealth and Lifestyles of the Older Population in England: The 2002 English Longitudinal Study of Ageing*. London: Institute for Fiscal Studies: 301–16 and Annex 8.1: 317–55.

Hyde, M., Wiggins, R.D., Higgs, P. and Blane, D.B. (2003) A measure of quality of life in early old age: the theory, development and properties of a needs satisfaction model (CASP-19), *Aging and Mental Health*, 7(3): 186–94.

Inglehart, R. (1997) *Modernization and Postmodernization: Cultural, Economic and Political Change in 43 Societies*. Princeton, NJ: Princeton University Press.

Iredell, H., Grenade, L., Boldy, D. et al. (2003) *Coping with Loneliness and Social Isolation in Later Life: A Pilot Study*. Perth, WA: Freemasons Centre for Research into Aged Care Services, Curtin University of Technology.

Janevic, M., Gjonaa, E. and Hyde, M. (2003) Physical and social environment, in M. Marmot, J. Banks, R. Blundell, C. Lessof and J. Nazroo (eds) *Health, Wealth and Lifestyles of the Older Population in England: The 2002 English Longitudinal Study of Ageing*. London: Institute for Fiscal Studies: 167–79 and Annex 5.1: 181–206.

Jarrett, P.G., Rockwood, K., Carver, D. et al. (1995) Illness presentation in elderly patients, *Archives of Internal Medicine*, 155: 1060–4.

Jenkins, C.L. (1997) Women, work and caregiving: how do these roles affect women's well-being? *Journal of Women and Aging*, 9: 27–45.

Jerrome, D. (1997) Ties that bind, in A. Walker (ed.) *The New Generational Contract: Intergenerational Relations, Old Age and Welfare*. London: University College London Press: 81–99.

Kahn, R.L. and Antonucci, T.C. (1980) Convoys over the life course: attachment roles and social support, in P.B. Baltes and O.G. Brim (eds) *Life-span development and behavior*. New York: Academic Press: 253–86.

Kahneman, D., Frederickson, B.L., Schreiber, C.A. and Redelmeier, D.A. (1993) When more pain is preferred to less: adding a better end, *Psychological Science*, 4: 401–5.

Kastenbaum, R.J. (1988) 'Safe death' in the postmodern world, in A. Gilmore and S. Gilmore (eds) *A Safer Death*. New York: Plenum.

Katbamna, S. and Bakta, P. with Parker, G., Ahmad, W. and Baker, R. (1998) *Experiences and Needs of Carers from the South Asian Communities*. Leicester: Nuffield Community Care Studies Unit.

Kaufman, S. (1998) Illness, biography and the interpretation of self following a stroke, *Journal of Aging Studies*, 2(3): 217–27.

Kaufman, S.R. (1986) *The Ageless Self: Sources of Meaning in Late Life*. Madison, WI: University of Wisconsin Press.

Kellaher, L. (2002) Is genuine choice a reality? The range and adequacy of living arrangements for older people, in K. Sumner (ed.) *Our Homes, Our*

Lives: Choice in Later Life Living Arrangement. London: CPA/Housing Corporation: 36–59.

Kershaw, C., Chivite-Matthews, N., Thomas, C. and Aust, R. (2001) *The 2001 British Crime Survey: First Results, England and Wales.* Home Office Statistical Bulletin 18/01. London: Stationery Office.

King, M., Speck, P. and Thomas, A. (2001) The Royal Free Interview for Spiritual and Religious Beliefs: development and validation of a self-report version, *Psychological Medicine*, 31: 1015–23.

Kitwood, T. (1997) *Dementia Reconsidered: The Person Comes.* Buckingham: Open University Press.

Kruk, E. (1995) Grandparent–grandchild contact loss: findings from a study of 'Grandparents Rights' members, *Canadian Journal on Aging*, 14: 737–54.

Kubler-Ross, E. (1990) *On Death and Dying.* London: Routledge.

Kubovy, M. (1999) On the pleasures of the mind, in D. Kahneman, E. Diener and N. Schwarz (eds) *Well-Being: The Foundations of Hedonic Psychology.* New York: Russell Sage Foundation: 134–54.

Kuh, D. and Ben-Shlomo, Y. (1997) Introduction: A life course approach to the aetiology of adult chronic disease, in D. Kuh and Y. Ben-Shlomo (eds) *A Life Course Approach to Chronic Disease Epidemiology.* Oxford: Oxford Medical Publications: 3–14.

Laslett, P. (1991) *A Fresh Map of Life: The Emergence of the Third Age.* Cambridge, MA: Harvard University Press.

Laws, G. (1984) Contested meanings, the built environment and aging in place, *Environment and Planning*, 26: 1787–802.

Lawton, M.P. (1975) The Philadelphia Geriatric Center Morale Scale: a revision, *Journal of Gerontology*, 30(1): 85–9.

Lawton, M.P. (1980) *Environment and Aging.* Monterey, CA: Brooks/Cole Publishing.

Lefebvre, H. (1991) *The Production of Space.* Oxford: Blackwell.

Lefebvre, H. (1994) *Everyday Life in the Modern World.* Trans. Sacha Rabinovitch. New Brunswick: Transaction Publishers.

Lillard, L.A. and Waite, L.J. (1995) Till death do us part: marital disruption and mortality, *American Journal of Sociology*, 100: 1131–56.

Lipsky, M. (1971) Social scientists and the AOL Commission, *Annals of the American Academy of Political and Social Science*, 394: 72–83.

Lund, D.A., Caserta, M.S. and Dimond, M. (1993) The course of spousal bereavement in later life, in M.S. Stroebe, W. Stroebe and R.O. Hansson *Handbook of Bereavement: Theory, Research and Intervention*. Cambridge: Cambridge University Press.

MacDonald, B. and Rich, C. (1984) *Look Me in the Eye*. London: The Women's Press.

Macintyre, S., Kearns, A. and Ellaway, A. (2000) *Housing Tenure and Car Ownership: Why Do They Predict Health and Longevity?* Final report of ESRC grant L12851017, ESRC, Swindon.

Marks, S. (1977) Multiple roles and role strain: some notes on human energy, time and commitment, *American Sociological Review*, 42: 921–36.

Markus, H. and Nurius, P. (1986) Possible selves, *American Psychologist*, 41: 954–69.

Marmot, M., Banks, J., Blundell, R., Lessof, C. and Nazroo, J. (eds) (2003) *Health, Wealth and Lifestyles of the Older Population in England: The 2002 English Longitudinal Study of Ageing*. London: Institute for Fiscal Studies.

Martin, T.L. and Doka, K.J. (1998) *Men Don't Cry . . . Women Do: Transcending Gender Stereotypes of Grief*. London: Brunner Mazell.

Matheson, J. and Summerfield, C. (eds) (1999) *Social Focus on Older People*. London: The Stationery Office.

McCormick, K. (2003) Social isolation in later life. Unpublished MSc thesis, St George's Hospital Medical School, University of London.

McKee, K.J. (1998) The Body Drop: a framework for understanding recovery from falls in older people, *Generations Review*, 8: 11–12.

McKee, K.J., Houston, D.M. and Barnes, S. (2002) Methods for assessing quality of life and well-being in frail older people, *Psychology and Health*, 17(6): 737–51.

McKee, K., Wilson, F., Elford, H., Goudie, F., Chung, M.C., Bolton, G. and Hinchliff, S. (2002) *Evaluating the Impact of Reminiscence on the Quality of Life of Older People*. GO Findings 8, Sheffield: Growing Older Programme, University of Sheffield.

McKevitt, C., Coshall, C., Mold, F., Tilling, K. and Wolfe, C. (2003) Explaining Inequalities in Health and Health Care after Stroke. Report to the Department of Health. London: King's College, Department of Public Health Sciences.

McMullin, J.A. (2000) Diversity and the state of sociological aging theory, *Gerontologist*, 40(5): 517–30.

Mead, G.H. (1934) *Mind, Self and Society from the Standpoint of a Social Behaviorist*. Chicago: University of Chicago Press.

Mendola, W.F. and Pelligrini, R.V. (1979) Quality of life and coronary artery bypass surgery patients, *Social Science and Medicine*, 13A: 457–61.

Midwinter, E. (1992) *Leisure: New Opportunities in the Third Age. The Carnegie Inquiry into the Third Age*. London: Carnegie Trust.

Mills, M. (1997) Narrative identity and dementia: a study of emotion and narrative in older people with dementia, *Ageing and Society*, 17: 673–98.

Mills, M. and Coleman, P. (1994) Nostalgic memories in dementia: a case study, *International Journal on Aging and Human Development*, 38(3): 203–19.

Mills, M. (2002) Supporting beliefs in later life: a challenge to churches and other faith communities. Paper presented at the Annual Conference for PSIGE, June 2002.

Minkler, M. and Estes, C. (1984) (eds) *Readings in the Political Economy of Aging*. New York: Baywood.

Modood, T., Berthoud, R., Lakey, J., Nazroo, J., Smith, P., Virdee, S. and Beishon, S. (1997) *Ethnic Minorities in Britain: Diversity and Disadvantage*, London: Policy Studies Institute.

Montgomery, S., Berney, L. and Blane, D. (2000) Pre-pubertal growth and blood pressure in early old age, *Archives of Disease in Childhood*, 82: 358–63.

Moriarty, J. and Butt, J. (2004) Social support and ethnicity in old age, in A. Walker and C.H. Hennessy (eds) *Growing Older: Quality of Life in Old Age*. Maidenhead: Open University Press: 167–87.

Myers, D.G. (2000) The funds, friends and faith of happy people, *American Psychologist*, 55(1): 56–67.

Myers, D.G. and Diener, E. (1996) The pursuit of happiness, *Scientific American*, 274: 54–6.

Myles, J. and Quadagno, J. (eds) (1993) *States, Labor Markets and the Future of Old-Age Policy*. Philadelphia, PA: Temple University Press.

Nazroo, J., Bajekal, M., Blane, D., Grewal, I. and Lewis, J. (2003) *Ethnic Inequalities in Quality of Life at Older Ages: Subjective and Objective Components*. GO Findings 11, Sheffield: Growing Older Programme, University of Sheffield.

Netz, Y. and Ben-Sira, D. (1993) Attitudes of young people, adults and older adults from three generation families toward the concepts 'ideal person', 'youth', 'adult' and 'old person', *Educational Gerontology*, 19: 607–21.

Neugarten, B.L., Havighurst, R.J. and Tobin, S.S. (1961) The measurement of life satisfaction, *Journal of Gerontology*, 16: 134–43.

Nolan, M., Davies, S. and Grant, G. (2001) Introduction: the changing face of health and social care, in M. Nolan, S. Davies and G. Grant (eds) *Working with Older People and Their Families*. Buckingham: Open University Press: 4–18.

Öberg, P. and Tornstam, L. (1999) Body images among men and women of different ages, *Ageing and Society*, 19: 629–44.

OECD (1988) *Reforming Public Pensions*. Paris: OECD.

Office for National Statistics (2000) *Family Spending: A Report on the 1999–2000 Family Expenditure Survey*. London: The Stationery Office.

OPCS (1991) *Standard Occupational Classification*. Vols 1–3. London: HMSO.

Owen, T. and Bell, L. (2004) *Quality of Life in Older Age; Messages from the Growing Older Programme*. London: Help the Aged in conjunction with ESRC.

Parkes, C.M. (1996) *Bereavement: Studies of Grief in Adult Life*, 3rd edn. Harmondsworth: Penguin.

Peace, S., Holland, C. and Kellaher, L. (2003) *Environment and Identity in Later Life: a cross-setting study*. GO Findings 18, Sheffield: Growing Older Programme, University of Sheffield.

Penning, M.J. (1998) In the middle: parental caregiving in the context of other roles, *Journal of Gerontology: Social Sciences*, 53B: S188–97.

Peterson, C. (1999) Personal control and well-being, in D. Kahneman, E. Diener and N. Schwarz (eds) *Well-Being: The Foundations of Hedonic Psychology*. New York: Russell Sage Foundation: 288–301.

Phillipson, C. (1997) Social relationships in later life: a review of the research literature, *International Journal of Geriatric Psychology*, 12: 505–12.

Phillipson, C., Bernard, M., Phillips, J. and Ogg, J. (1999) Older people's experience of community life: patterns of neighbouring in three urban areas, *Sociological Review*, 47(4): 715–43.

Phillipson, C., Bernard, M., Phillips, J. and Ogg, J. (2001) *Family and Community Life of Older People*. London: Routledge.

Porter, R. (1997) *The Greatest Benefit to Mankind: A Medical History of Humanity from Antiquity to the Present*. London: HarperCollins Publishers.

Pound, P., Gompertz, P. and Ebrahim, S. (1998) Illness in the context of older age: the case of stroke, *Sociology of Health & Illness*, 20(4): 489–506.

Power, C., Stansfeld, S.A., Matthew, S., Manor, O. and Hope, S. (2002) Childhood and adulthood risk factors for socio-economic differentials in psychological distress: evidence from the 1958 birth cohort, *Social Science and Medicine*, 55: 1989–2004.

Quereshi, H. and Walker, A. (1989) *The Caring Relationship: Elderly People and their Families*. London: Macmillan.

Reboussin, B.A., Rejeski, W.J., Martin, K.A. et al. (2000) Correlates of body satisfaction with body function and body appearance in middle- and older aged adults: the Activity Counseling Trial (ACT), *Psychology and Health*, 15: 239–54.

Reid, J. and Hardy, M. (1999) Multiple roles and well-being among midlife women: testing role strain and role enhancement theories, *Journal of Gerontology: Social Sciences*, 54B: S329–38.

Reitzes, D.C., Mutran, E.J. and Fernandez, M.E. (1996) Does retirement hurt well-being? Factors influencing self-esteem and depression among retirees and workers, *The Gerontologist*, 36: 649–56.

Reker, G.T. (1996) *Manual of the Life Attitude Profile-Revised (LAP-R)*. Peterborough, ON: Student Psychologists Press.

Renwick, R. and Brown, I. (1996) Being, belonging, becoming: the Centre for Health Promotion model of quality of life, in R. Renwick, I. Brown and M. Nagler (eds) *Quality of Life in Health Promotion and Rehabilitation: Conceptual Approaches, Issues and Applications*. Thousand Oaks, CA: Sage: 75–88.

Ritchie, J. and Spencer, L. (1993) Qualitative data analysis for applied policy research, in A. Bryman and R. Burgess (eds) *Analysing Qualitative Data*. London: Routledge: 173–94.

Robertson, I., Warr, P., Butcher, V., Callinan, M. and Bardzil, P. (2003) *Older People's Experience of Paid Employment: Participation and Quality of Life*. GO Findings 14, Sheffield: Growing Older Programme, University of Sheffield.

Rockwood, K., Stadnyk, K., MacKnight, C. et al. (1999) A brief clinical instrument to classify frailty in elderly people, *Lancet*, 353: 205–6.

Rosenthal, C.J., Martin-Matthews, A. and Matthews, S.H. (1996) Caught in the middle? Occupancy in multiple roles and help to parents in a national probability sample of Canadian adults, *Journal of Gerontology: Social Sciences*, 51B: S274–83.

Ross, C.E. and Drentea, P. (1998) Consequences of retirement activities for distress and sense of personal control, *Journal of Health and Social Behaviour*, 39: 317–34.

Ross, M., Eyman, A. and Kishchuck, N. (1986) Determinants of subjective well-being, in J.M. Olson, C.P. Herman and M. Zanna (eds) *Relative Deprivation and Social Comparison*. Hillsdale, NJ: Erlbaum.

Rowe, J.W. and Kahn, R.L. (1987) Human aging: usual and successful, *Science*, 237: 143–9.

Rowe, J.W. and Kahn, R.L. (1997) Successful aging, *The Gerontologist*, 37(4): 433–40.

Rowles, G.D. (1978) *Prisoners of Space? Exploring the Geographical Experience of Older People*. Boulder, CO: Westview Press.

Rowles, G.D. (2000) Habituation and being in place, *Occupational Therapy Journal of Research*, 20(1): 52S–67S.

Rubenstein, R.L. (1989) The home environment of older people: a description of psychosocial processes linking person to place, *Journal of Gerontology*, 44: S45–S53.

Runyan, W.M. (1980) The life satisfaction chart: perceptions of the course of subjective experience, *International Journal of Aging and Human Development*, 11: 45–64.

Ryan, R.M. and Deci, E.L. (2000) Self-determination theory and the facilitation of intrinsic motivation, social developmentand well-being, in M.E.P. Seligman and M. Csikszentmihalyi (eds) *Special Issue on Happiness, Excellence and Optimal Human Functioning. American Psychologist*, 55: 68–78.

Ryan, R.M. and Deci, E.L. (2001) On happiness and human potential: a review of research on hedonic and eudaimonic well-being, *Annual Review of Psychology*, 52: 141–66.

Ryder, N.B. (1985) The cohort as a concept in the study of social change, in W.M. Mason and S.E Fienberg (eds) *Cohort Analysis in Social Research: Beyond the Identification Problem*. New York: Springer-Verlag: 9–44.

Ryff, C.D. and Singer, B. (1998) The contours of positive human health, *Psychological Inquiry*, 9: 1–28.

Ryff, C.D. and Singer, B. (2000) Interpersonal flourishing: a positive health agenda for the new millennium, *Personality and Social Psychology Review*, 4: 30–44.

Salthouse, T.A., Berish, D.E. and Miles, J.D. (2002) The role of cognitive stimulation on the relations between age and cognitive functioning, *Psychology and Aging*, 14: 483–506.

Sapp, S. (1987) An alternative Christian view of aging, *Journal of Religion and Aging*, 4(1): 69–85.

Sarbin, T.R. (1986) The narrative as a root metaphor for psychology, in T.R. Sarbin (ed.) *Narrative Psychology: The Storied Nature of Human Conduct*. New York: Praeger.

Scase, R. and Scales, J. (2000) *Fit and Fifty*. Swindon: ESRC.

Schaie, K.M. and Willis, S.L. (2002) *Adult Development and Aging*. Upper Saddle River, NJ: Prentice Hall.

Scharf, T., Phillipson, C. and Smith, A.E. (2004) Poverty and social exclusion: growing older in deprived urban neighbourhoods, in A. Walker and C. Hagan Hennessy (eds) *Growing Older: Quality of Life in Old Age*. Buckingham: Open University Press.

Scharf, T., Phillipson, C., Kingston, P. and Smith, A.E. (2000) Social exclusion and ageing, *Education and Ageing*, 16(3): 303–20.

Scharf, T., Phillipson, C., Smith, A.E. and Kingston, P. (2002) *Growing Older in Socially Deprived Areas: Social Exclusion in Later Life*. London: Help the Aged.

Scharf, T., Phillipson, C., Smith, A.E. and Kingston, P. (2003) *Older People in Deprived Neighbourhoods: Social Exclusion and Quality of Life in Old Age*. GO Findings 19, Sheffield: Growing Older Programme, University of Sheffield.

Scharf, T. and Smith, A.E. (2004) Older people in urban neighbourhoods: addressing the risk of social exclusion in later life, in C. Phillipson, G. Allan and D. Morgan (eds) *Social Networks and Social Exclusion*. Aldershot: Ashgate: 162–79.

Schwartz, N. (1987) *Mood as Information*. Heidelberg: Springer-Verlag.

Schwartz, N. and Clore, G.L. (1983) Mood, misattribution and judgments of well-being: informative and directive functions of affective states, *Journal of Personality and Social Psychology*, 45: 513–23.

Schwartz, N. and Strack, F. (1991) Context effects in attitude surveys: applying cognitive theory to social research, in W. Stroebe and M. Hewstone (eds) *European Review of Social Psychology*, Vol. 2. Chichester: John Wiley.

Schwartz, N., Strack, F. and Mai, H.P. (1991) Assimilation and contrast effects in part-whole question sequences: a conversational logic hypothesis, *Public Opinion Quarterly*, 55: 2–23.

Sheldon, J.H. (1948) *The Social Medicine of Old Age*. Oxford: Oxford University Press.

Shin, D.C. and Johnson, D.M. (1978) Avowed happiness as an overall assessment of the quality of life, *Social Indicators Research*, 5: 475–92.

Sidell, M. (1995) *Health in Old Age*. Buckingham: Open University Press.

Sidorenko, A. and Walker, A. (2004) The Madrid International Plan of Action on Ageing: from conception to implementation, *Ageing and Society*, 24: 147–65.

Sieber, S. (1974) Toward a theory of role accumulation, *American Sociological Review*, 39: 567–78.

Singh-Manoux, A., Clarke, P. and Marmot, M. (2002) Multiple measures of socio-economic position and psychosocial health: proximal and distal measures, *International Journal of Epidemiology*, 31: 1192–9.

Smith, A.E. (2001) Defining quality of life, *Growing Older Programme Newsletter*, 2: 3.

Smith, A.E. (2000) Quality of life: a review, *Education and Ageing*, 15(3): 419–35.

Smith, A.E., Phillipson, C. and Scharf, T. (2002) *Social Capital: Concepts, Measures and the Implications for Urban Communities*, Working Paper 9. Keele: Centre for Social Gerontology, Keele University.

Smith, T.W. (1979) Happiness, *Social Psychology Quarterly*, 42: 18–30.

Social Exclusion Unit (1998) *Bringing Britain Together: A National Strategy for Neighbourhood Renewal*. London: Stationery Office.

Social Services Inspectorate (1998) *They Look After Their Own, Don't They? Inspection of Community Care Services for Black and Ethnic Minority Older People*. London: Department of Health.

Speck, P. (*in press*) Dementia and spiritual care, in G.M.M. Jones and B.M.L. Miesen *Care Giving in Dementia: Research and Application*, vol. 4. London: Routledge.

Spitze, G. and Logan, J.R. (1990) More evidence on women (and men) in the middle, *Research on Aging*, 12: 182–98.

Spitze, G., Logan, J.R., Joseph, G. and Lee, E. (1994) Middle generation roles and the well-being of men and women, *Journal of Gerontology: Social Sciences*, 49: S107–16.

Stephen, A. and Raftery, J. (eds) (1994) *Health Care Needs Assessment*, vol 1. Oxford: Radcliffe Medical Press.

Stevens, T., Wilde, D., Paz, S., Ahmedzai, S., Rawson, A. and Wragg, D. (2004) Palliative care research protocols: a special case for ethical review? *Palliative Medicine*, 17: 482–90.

Strack, F., Martin, L.L and Schwartz, N. (1988) Priming and communication: social determinants of information use in judgments of life satisfaction, *European Journal of Social Psychology*, 18, 429–42.

Strack, F., Schwartz, N., Chassein, B., Kern, D. and Wagner, D. (1990) The salience of comparison standards and the activation of social norms: consequences for judgments of happiness and their communication, *British Journal of Social Psychology*, 29: 303–14.

Stroebe, M.S., Stroebe, W. and Hansson, R.O. (1993) *Handbook of Bereavement: Theory, Research and Intervention*. Cambridge: Cambridge University Press.

Stroebe, W. and Stroebe, M.S. (1987) *Bereavement and Health: The Psychological and Physical Consequences of Parental Loss*. Cambridge: Cambridge University Press.

Summerfield, C. and Babb, P. (eds) (2004) *Social Trends No. 34*. London: The Stationery Office.

Swan, G.E., Dame, A. and Carmelli, D. (1991) Involuntary retirement, type A behavior and current functioning in elderly men: 27-year follow-up of the Western Collaborative Group Study, *Psychology and Aging*, 6: 384–91.

Sweeting, H.N. and Gilhooly, M.L.M. (1992) Doctor, am I dead? Social death in modern societies, *Omega: The Journal of Thanatology*, 24(4): 255–73.

Tester, S., Hubbard, G. and Downs, M. (2001) Defining quality of life among frail older people. *Growing Older Programme Newsletter*, 2: 7.

Tester, S., Hubbard, G., Downs, M., MacDonald, C. and Murphy, J. (2003) *Exploring Perceptions of Quality of Life of Frail Older People During and After their Transition to Institutional Care*. GO Findings 24, Sheffield: Growing Older Programme, University of Sheffield.

The Royal Commission on Long-Term Care (1999) *With Respect to Old Age*, CM 4192–1. London: The Stationery Office.

Thompson, L. and Walker, A. (1987) Mothers as mediators of intimacy between grandmothers and their young adult granddaughters, *Family Relation*, 36: 72–7.

Thompson, P., Itzin, C. and Abendstern, M. (1990) *I Don't Feel Old: The Experience of Later Life*. Oxford: Oxford University Press.

Tijhuis, M.A., Jong Gierveld, J. de, Festiens, E.J. and Kromhout, D. (1999) Changes in and factors related to loneliness in men: the Lutphen Elderly Study, *Age and Ageing*, 28(5): 491–5.

Townsend, P. (1962) *The Last Refuge*. London: Routledge and Kegan Paul.

Townsend, P. (1968) Isolation and loneliness, in E. Shanas, P. Townsend, D. Wedderburn et al. (eds) *Old People in Three Industrial Societies*. London: Routledge & Kegan Paul: 258–88.

Tsang, E.Y.L., Liamputtong, P. and Pierson, J. (2004) The views of older Chinese people in Melbourne about their quality of life, *Ageing and Society*, 24(1): 51–74.

Tunstall, J. (1966) *Old and Alone*. London: Routledge and Kegan Paul.

Turner, B.S. (1995) Ageing and identity: some reflections on the somatization of the self, in M. Featherstone and A. Wernick (eds) *Images of Ageing. Cultural Representations of Later Life*. London: Routledge: 245–62.

Ungerson, C. (1999) Personal assistants and disabled people: an examination of a hybrid form of work and care, *Work, Employment and Society*, 13(4): 483–600.

Unsworth, K., McKee, K.J. and Mulligan, C. (2001) When does old age begin? The role of attitudes in age parameter placement, *Social Psychological Review*, 3(2): 5–15.

Utz, R., Carr, D., Nesse, R. and Wortman, C. (2002) The effect of widowhood on older adult's social participation: an evaluation of activity, disengagement and continuity theories, *The Gerontologist*, 42(4): 522–33.

Verbrugge, L.M. (1983) Multiple roles and physical health of women and men. *Journal of Health and Social Behavior*, 24: 16–30.

Victor, C.R., Bowling, A., Bond, J. and Scambler, S. (2003) *Loneliness, Social Isolation and Living Alone in Later Life*, ESRC Growing Older Programme Findings, No 17, University of Sheffield.

Victor, C.R., Scambler, S., Bond, J. and Bowling, A. (2000) Being alone in later life: loneliness, isolation and living alone in later life, *Reviews in Clinical Gerontology*, 10(4): 407–17.

Victor, C.R., Scambler, S., Bond, J. and Bowling, A. (2001) Loneliness in later life: preliminary findings from the Growing Older Project, *Quality in Ageing*, 3(1): 34–41.

Victor, C.R., Scambler, S., Shah, S., Cook, D.G., Harris, T., Rink, E. and Wilde, S. de (2002) Has loneliness among older people increased? An investigation into variations between cohorts, *Ageing and Society*, 22: 1–13.

Vitz, P.C. (1990) The use of stories in moral development: new psychological reasons for an old education method, *American Psychologist*, 45: 709–20.

Voyandoff, P. and Donnelly, B.W. (1999) Multiple roles and psychological distress: the intersection of the paid worker, spouse and parent roles with the role of the adult child, *Journal of Marriage and the Family*, 61: 725–38.

Walker, A. (1980) The social creation of poverty and dependency in old age, *Journal of Social Policy*, 9(1): 45–75.

Walker, A. (1981) Towards a political economy of old age, *Ageing and Society*, 1(1): 73–94.

Walker, A. (1990) The economic 'burden' of ageing and the prospect of inter-generational conflict, *Ageing and Society*, 10(4): 377–96.

Walker, A. (ed.) (1997a) *The New Generational Contract*. London: UCL Press.

Walker, A. (1997b) *Combating Age Barriers in Employment*. Luxembourg: Office for Official Publications of the European Communities.

Walker, A. (2001) Introduction to the Second Newsletter of the Growing Older Programme: Defining Quality of Life, *Growing Older Programme Newsletter*, 2: 1.

Walker, A. (2002) A strategy for active ageing, *International Social Security Review*, 55(1): 121–40.

Walker, A. (2004) Introducing the Growing Older Programme on extending quality life, in A. Walker and C.H. Hennessy (eds) *Growing Older: Quality of Life in Old Age*. Maidenhead: Open University Press.

Walker, A. (2004) The ESRC Growing Older Research Programme 1999–2004, *Ageing and Society*, 24: 657–75.

Walker, A. (ed.) (2005a) *Growing Older in Europe*. Maidenhead: Open University Press.

Walker, A. (2005b) Re-examining the political economy of ageing: understanding the structure/agency tension, in J. Baars, D. Dannefer, C. Phillipson and A. Walker (eds) *Ageing, Globalisation and Inequality: The New Critical Gerontology*. New York: Baywood.

Walker, A. and Deacon, B. (2003) Economic globalisation and policies on ageing, *Journal of Societal and Social Policy*, 2(2): 1–18.

Walker, A. and Hennessy, C.H. (2003) *Growing Older Programme Project Summaries*. Swindon: Economic and Social Research Council.

Walker, A. and Hagan Hennessy, C.H. (eds) (2004) *Growing Older: Quality of Life in Old Age*. Maidenhead: Open University Press.

Walker, A. and Maltby, T. (1997) *Ageing Europe*. Buckingham: Open University Press.

Walker, A. and Martimo, K. (2000) Researching quality of life in old age, *Quality in Ageing: Policy, Practice and Research*, 1(1): 8–14.

Walker, A. and Naegele, G. (eds) (1999) *The Politics of Ageing in Europe*. Buckingham: Open University Press.

Walker, A. and Taylor, P. (1998) *Combating Age Barriers in Employment: Portfolio of Good Practice*. Dublin: European Foundation.

Walker, A., O'Brien, M., Traynor, J., Fox, K., Goddard, E. and Foster, K. (eds) (2003) *Living in Britain: Results from the 2001 General Household Survey. Supplementary Report: People Aged 65 and Over*. http://www.statistics.gov.uk/lib2001/section3730.html (accessed 17 May 2004).

Walter, T. (1996) A new model of grief: bereavement and biography, *Mortality*, 1: 7–25.

Walter, T. (1999) *On Bereavement*. Buckingham: Open University Press.

Warr, P.B. (1987) *Work, Unemployment and Mental Health*. Oxford: Oxford University Press.

Warr, P.B., Butcher, V. and Robertson, I.T. (2004) Activity and psychological well-being in older people, *Aging and Mental Health*, 8: 172–83.

Warr, P.B., Butcher, V., Robertson, I.T. and Callinan, M. (2004) Older people's well-being as a function of employment, retirement, environmental characteristics and role preference, *British Journal of Psychology* (in press).

Warr, P.B., Jackson, P.R. and Banks, M. H. (1988) Unemployment and mental health: some British studies, *Journal of Social Issues*, 44: 47–68.

Waterman, A.S. (1993) Two conceptions of happiness: contrasts of personal expressiveness and hedonic enjoyment, *Journal of Personality and Social Psychology*, 64: 678–91.

Weber, M. (1968) *Economy and Society*. New York: Bedminster Press.

Weiss, C. (1980) Knowledge creep and decision accretion, *Knowledge: Creation, Diffusion, Utilisation*, 1(3): 381–404.

Weiss, C. (1986) Research and policy-making: a limited partnership, in F. Heller (ed.) *The Use and Abuse of Social Science*. London: Sage.

Welin, L., Tibblin, G., Svardsudd, K. et al. (1985) Prospective study of social influences on mortality: the study of men born in 1913 and 1923, *Lancet*, 1 (8434): 915–18.

Wenger, G.C. (1983) Loneliness: a problem of measurement, in D. Jerrome (ed.) *Ageing in Modern Society*. Beckenham, Kent: Croom Helm: 145–67.

Wenger, G.C. (1984) *The Supportive Network*. London: George Allen and Unwin.

Wenger, G.C. and Burholt, V. (2004) Changes in levels of social isolation and loneliness among older people in rural Wales – a 20 year longitudinal study, *Canadian Journal on Ageing*, 23, 115–27.

Wenger, G.C., Davies, R., Shahtahmesebi, S. and Scott, A. (1996) Social isolation and loneliness in old age: review and model refinement, *Ageing and Society*, 16: 333–58.

WHO (2001a) *Active Ageing: From Evidence to Action*. Geneva: World Health Organization.

WHO (2001b) *Health and Ageing: A Discussion Paper*. Geneva: World Health Organization.

Wiggins, R., Higgs, P., Hyde, M. and Blane, D. (2004) Quality of life in the third age: key predictors of the CASP-19 measure, *Ageing and Society*, 24: 693–708.

Willcocks, D., Peace, S. and Kellaher, L. (1987) *Private Lives in Public Places*. London: Tavistock Publications.

Williamson, J.D. and Fried, L.P. (1996) Characterization of older adults who attribute functional decrements to 'old age', *Journal of the American Geriatrics Society*, 44: 1429–34.

Wilson, G. (1994) Co-production and self-care: new approaches to managing community care services for older people, *Social Policy and Administration*, 28(3): 236–50.

Wilson, R.S., Mendes de Leon, D.F., Barnes, L.L. et al. (2002) Participation in cognitively stimulating activities and risk of incident Alzheimer disease, *Journal of the American Medical Association*, 288: 2271–81.

Woodhouse, K.W., Wynne, H., Baillie, S. et al. (1988) Who are the frail elderly?, *Quarterly Journal of Medicine*, 68: 505–6.

Woods, B., Portnoy, S., Head, D. et al. (1992) Reminiscence and life review with persons with dementia: which way forward? in B.M.L. Miesen and G.M.M. Jones (eds) *Care-giving in Dementia*. London: Routledge: 139–61.

Worden, J.W. (2003) *Grief Counselling and Grief Therapy*, 3rd edn. Hove: Brunner-Routledge.

World Health Organization Quality of Life Group (1993) *Measuring Quality of Life: The Development of the World Health Organization Quality of Life Instrument (WHOQOL)*. Geneva: World Health Organization.

Wortman, C.B. and Silver, R.C. (1989) The myths of coping with loss, *Journal of Consulting Clinical Psychology*, 57: 349–57.

Wray, S. (2004) Women growing older: agency, ethnicity and culture, *Sociology*, 37(3): 511–27.

Yu, W.K. (2000) *Chinese Older People: A Need for Social Inclusion in Two Communities*. York: Joseph Rowntree Foundation.

Index

Related books from Open University Press

Purchase from www.openup.co.uk or order through your local bookseller

GROWING OLDER
QUALITY OF LIFE IN OLD AGE

Alan Walker and Catherine Hagan Hennessy

This volume introduces the work of the Economic and Social Research Council (ESRC) funded Growing Older Programme (1999-2004) and provides a showcase for the other volumes in the series. It focuses on ways in which quality of life can be extended for older people and offers short research-based summaries of key findings on a variety of core topics with a major emphasis on the views of older people themselves.

Many of the leading names in social gerontology in the United Kingdom have contributed their findings, providing the most up-to-date and broad-ranging information available on quality of life in old age. Topics discussed include:

- Defining and measuring quality of life
- Inequalities in quality of life
- Technology and the built environment
- Healthy and active ageing
- Family and support networks
- Participation and grandparenthood

Growing Older is suitable for undergraduate and postgraduate students of social gerontology, sociology and social policy. It is of interest to professionals working with older people, including social workers, gerontology nurses and community support workers. There are also important findings for policy-makers.

Contributors:
Sara Arber; Madhavi Bajekal; David Blane; John Bond; Ann Bowling; Jabeer Butt; Lynda Clarke; Joanne Cook; Kate Davidson; Murna Downs; Zahava Gabriel; Ini Grewal; Catherine Hagan Hennessey; Caroline Holland; Gill Hubbard; Leonie Kellaher; Charlotte MacDonald; Tony Maltby; Jo Moriarty; Joan Murphy; James Nazroo; Sheila M. Peace; Chris Phillipson; Ceridwen Roberts; Sasha Scambler; Thomas Scharf; Allison Smith; Susan Tester; Christina Victor; Alan Walker; Lorna Warren.

Contents:
Contributors – Preface – Introducing the Growing Older Programme on extending quality of life – Quality of life in old age from the perspectives of older people – Ethnic inequalities – Environment, identity and old age: Quality of life or a life of quality? – Poverty and social exclusion: Growing older in deprived urban neighbourhoods – Loneliness in later life – Older men: Their health behaviours and partnership status – A participatory approach to older women's quality of life – Social support and ethnicity in old age – The meaning of grandparenthood, and its contribution to the quality of life of older people – Frailty and institutional life – Conclusion – Bibliography – Index.

c.280pp   0 335 21507 6 (Paperback)   0 335 21508 4 (Hardback)

GROWING OLDER
GROWING OLDER IN EUROPE

Alan Walker

Growing Older in Europe is a companion volume to the other books in the Growing Older series and provides the first comparative European perspective on ageing. The comparisons demonstrate that although similar quality of later life issues are faced by older people in different European Union countries, the policy and service contexts are significantly different, as are the research traditions.

Based on systematic reviews of evidence from the United Kingdom, Germany, Italy, the Netherlands and Sweden, the book provides a unique resource for anyone interested in the rapidly growing field of ageing.

Written by prominent experts, the research evidence highlights topics such as:

- physical and mental health
- the environments of ageing
- employment and income
- family and support networks
- participation and social integration
- good practice in the promotion of quality of life

The book is key reading for specialists, including students, practitioners and policy makers, as well as lay people with an interest in the fields of social gerontology, sociology and social policy.

Contributors:
Lars Andersson, Beitske Bouwman, Kees Knipscheer, Giovanni Lamura, Annemarie Peters, Francesca Polverini, Monika Reichert, Carol Walker, Manuela Weidekamp-Maicher.

Contents:
Contributors – Preface – Quality of life in old age in Europe – Part I. Quality of life in old age: definitions, environments and socio-economic aspects – Germany: quality of life in old age I – Italy: quality of life in old age I – The Netherlands: quality of life in old age I – Sweden: quality of life in old age I – The UK: quality of life in old age I – Part II. Quality of life in old age: participation, social support and subjective wellbeing – Germany: quality of life in old age II – Italy: quality of life in old age II – The Netherlands: quality of life in old age II – Sweden: quality of life in old age II – The UK: quality of life in old age II – References – Index

312pp   0 335 21513 0 (Paperback)   0 335 21514 9 (Hardback)

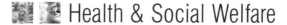  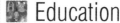

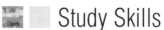

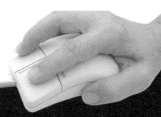